# Techniques for Nephropathology

Editors


**David E. Allen**
Lecturer in Histochemistry and Electron Microscopy
Department of Medical Technology
Queensland Institute of Technology
Brisbane, Australia

**John P. Dowling**
Deputy Directory
Anatomical Pathology
Royal Melbourne Hospital
Melbourne, Australia



CRC

**CRC Press, Inc.**
**Boca Raton, Florida**

**Library of Congress Cataloging in Publication Data**

Allen, David E.
Techniques for nephropathology.

Bibliography: p.
Includes index.
1. Kidneys — Biopsy. 2. Histology, Pathological — Technique. 3. Tissue culture.
I. Dowling, John P., joint author. II. Title.
[DNLM: 1. Kidney diseases — Diagnosis. 2. Kidney — Pathology. 3. Biopsy, Needle. WJ302 A425t]
RC903.9.A38 616.6′107583 80-22743
ISBN 0-8493-5791-8



Direct all inquiries to CRC Press, Inc., 2000 N.W. 24th Street, Boca Raton, Florida, 33431



International Standard Book Number 0-8493-5791-8

Library of Congress Card Number 80-22743
Printed in the United States

# PREFACE

It is our aim in this monograph to present techniques for the routine examination of renal tissue that are reliable and provide the maximum information for diagnosis. The methods described have provided consistently good results and to a varying degree represent a compilation of those previously advocated. Personal preference,* experience, and the quality of technical expertise usually determine which techniques are employed in an individual laboratory. Our methods were assembled after an extensive process of trial and error in applying different recommended techniques over recent years.

Accurate diagnosis of the renal biopsy remains the cornerstone of management of renal diseases and that diagnosis is often reached only after immunohistochemical and ultrastructural data have supplemented the light microscopic findings. Thus the techniques outlined cover, in the main, these three aspects of renal biopsy examination.

Morphological techniques, however, have not provided much of the basic information of the renal, especially glomerular, reaction to injury. In vitro glomerular culture promises much in this regard when applied to human tissue and the experimental situation. Thus we have included a chapter on this and related techniques by Associate Professor Robert Atkins and Associate Professor Eric Glasgow and their colleagues who commenced working in this field at Peince Henry's Hospital, Melbourne in 1972.

* Discussion in Strauss, J., Ed., *Pediatric Nephrology Vol. 4: Renal Failure — Current Concepts in Diagnosis and Management*, Garland ST PM Press, New York, 1978, 255.

## ACKNOWLEDGMENTS

We both wish to express our gratitude to the technicians who have prepared the sections for this work very skillfully and who responded to our constant demands magnificently. These personnel include Anselm Ambrose, Gary Chan, B. Sc. (who also provided figures), Peter Angus, and Gayle Sewell. Ian Birchall, Renal Pathology Technician at the Royal Melbourne Hospital, with his considerable experience, gave valuable assistance.

Dr. Michael Drake, Director of the Anatomical Pathology Department, Prince Henry's Hospital, Melbourne, provided us with the proper facilities with which to do this work and gave us both constant encouragement and guidance.

JPD wishes to especially thank a group of renal pathologists in Melbourne, Dr. David Davies, Professor Graeme Rayn, Dr. John Tange, and Dr. Joshua Xipell, for first stimulating his interest in renal pathology and maintaining it.

Associate Professor Eric Glasgow of the Department of Anatomy, Monash University first advised us on technical matters and recommended the use of Duboscq-Brasil fixation. He, together with Associate Professor Robert Atkins and Dr. Napier Thomson, respectively, Director and Deputy Director of the Nephrology Department at Prince Henry's Hospital, Melbourne, have provided enthusiastic support and encouragement over the years.

The manuscript has been carefully and skillfully typed by Mrs. Rosemary Goland and Ms. Maree Bearzatto. We are most grateful for their efforts.

**David E. Allen**
**John P. Dowling**

# EDITORS

**David Allen, Ph.D., A.R.A.C.I.,** is presently Senior Lecturer in Histotechnology and Histochemistry in the Department of Medical Technology at the Queensland Institute of Technology, Brisbane, Queensland, Australia. He was formerly at Prince Henry's Hospital in Melbourne as Senior Hospital Scientist in the Department of Anatomical Pathology.

After receiving his bachelor degree in Chemistry with First Class Honours from Birmingham University (England) in 1972, Dr. Allen moved to Canberra, Australia to carry out research into the design and use of organometallic complexes as stains for electron microscopy. He was awarded a Ph. D. from the Australian National University in 1976.

Dr. Allen has written or co-authored a number of articles on staining methods for electron microscopy and currently has research interests in the areas of electron microscopy and immunohistochemistry.

**John P. Dowling, M.B.B.S., F.R.C.P.A.,** is currently Deputy Director of the Department of Anatomical Pathology at The Royal Melbourne Hospital, Victoria, Australia. From 1974 to 1979 he was Staff Pathologist in the Department of Anatomical Pathology at Prince Henry's Hospital, Melbourne where he reported on general surgical pathology specimens. He was responsible for and specialized in nephropathology during this time.

At The Royal Melbourne Hospital, Dr. Dowling has pursued this interest in both the diagnostic and technical aspects of nephropathology.

# CONTRIBUTORS

**Robert C. Atkins**
Associate Professor of Medicine
Director, Department of Nephrology
Prince Henry's Hospital
Melbourne, Australia

**Eric Glasgow**
Associate Professor of Anatomy
Department of Anatomy
Monash University
Clayton, Victoria
Australia

**Wayne W. Hancock**
Research Fellow
Department of Medicine
Prince Henry's Hospital
Melbourne, Australia

# TABLE OF CONTENTS

Chapter 1

# COLLECTION AND INITIAL TREATMENT OF TISSUE

**David E. Allen and John P. Dowling**

## TABLE OF CONTENTS



## I. INTRODUCTION

Renal tissue is generally acquired by one of three methods, namely closed renal biopsy, open surgical biopsy, or at post-mortem. The biopsy procedures have been very adequately described elsewhere and will not be considered further. Open surgical biopsies if taken as a surgical wedge excision tend to provide mostly cortical tissue, and should deeper medullary tissue be required, a needle biopsy would appear to be more appropriate.

The amount of renal tissue provided for diagnostic purposes is critical. The diagnosis of diffuse renal diseases may require only a small amount of cortex and/or medulla to establish a diagnosis. Focal lesions, if minor, often require a very ample specimen for diagnosis. Thus, while one needle core containing cortex and medulla is often sufficient to provide specimens for light and electron microscopy and immunofluorescent examination, the acquisition of two adequate needle cores is preferable. In our experience the latter has not been associated with increased patient morbidity.

To ensure prompt and appropriate division of the tissue, a technician must attend the biopsy procedure. The use of a dissecting microscope can greatly assist both the clinician and the technician in the performance of a biopsy. Doubt often exists during a closed needle biopsy procedure as to whether renal tissue has been taken. The technician can more accurately determine what type of tissue (kidney, muscle, connective tissue, or fat) has been produced. With experience, naked-eye examination of the biopsy may suffice.

It is crucial that the technician identifies renal cortical and/or medullary tissue in the biopsy cores. Examination of the specimen should be carried out under moist conditions with the biopsy resting on saline-soaked cotton gauze in a Petri dish. It is also important to examine and divide the biopsy as quickly as possible to avoid delayed-fixation artifact for electron microscopy. The saline-soaked gauze will prevent the rapid dehydration that occurs with small-tissue biopsies. A strong indicent light used for examination of the specimen under the dissecting microscope will also dehydrate the specimen and should be avoided.

Glomeruli, particularly those that are congested, are just visible to the naked eye (Figure 1). The dissecting microscope aids identification of those that are not congested by showing them as small rounded discs that are seen particularly over the lateral margins of the biopsy. The cortical aspect of the biopsy often readily contrasts with the medulla which possesses parallel arrays of congested peritubular venules. However, the renal parenchyma obtained may not be congested in some instances making distinction

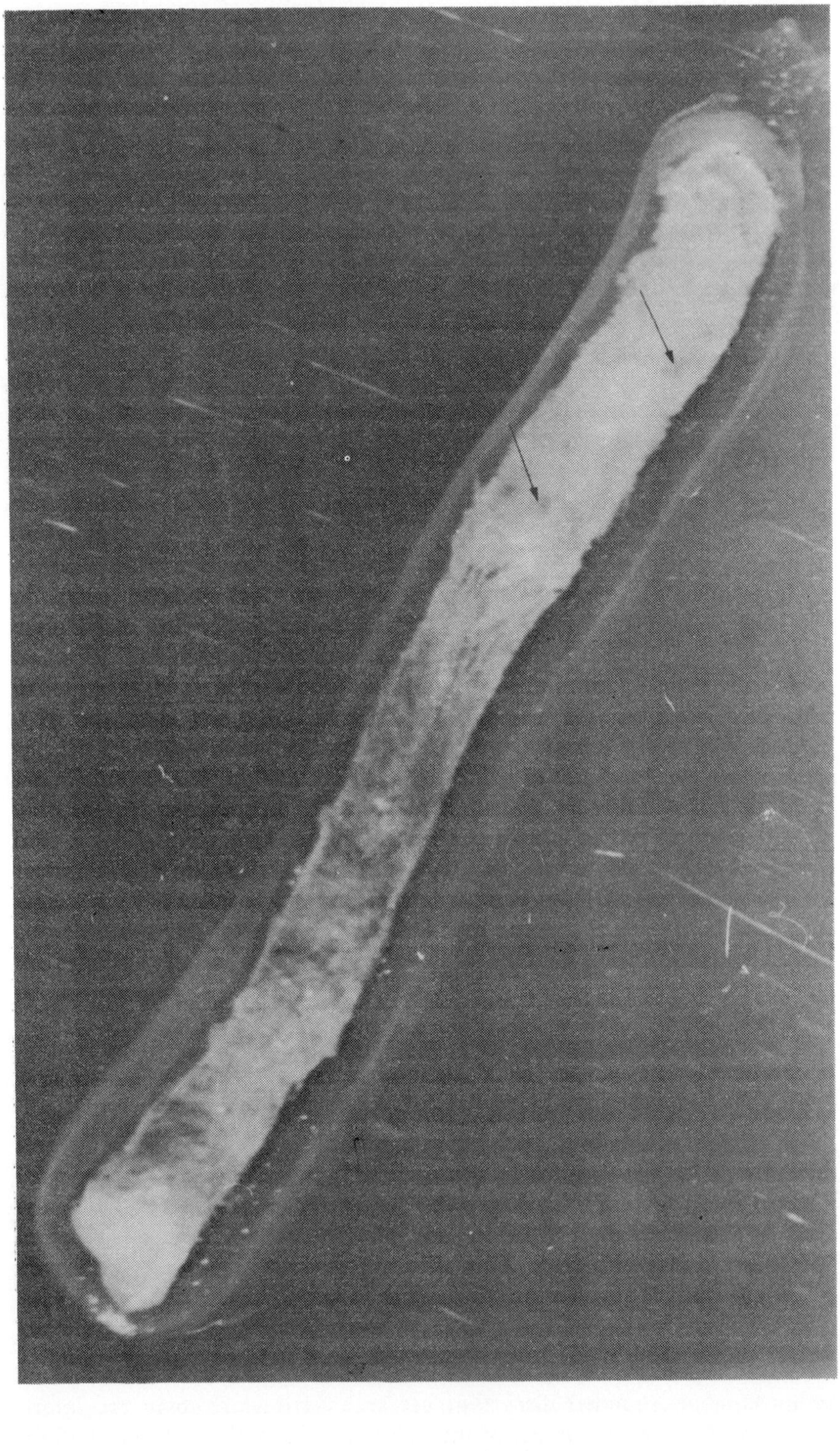

FIGURE 1. Renal needle core biopsy Glomeruli (arrowed) are just visible in the renal cortical tissue. (Original magnification $\times$ 10.)

between cortex and medulla very difficult; the presence of white fibrous capsular tissue may distinguish the cortical end of the biopsy in this circumstance.

If only one needle core comprising both cortex and medulla is available, it is dissected usually in one of two ways. From each end 1 $mm^3$ is taken and fixed for electron microscopy as soon as possible, ensuring that the small segments consist of renal parenchyma and not capsular or calyceal epithelial tissue. A further small section (1 to 2 mm in length) is taken from the cortical parenchyma for immunofluorescence. The remaining tissue consists of a variable amount of cortex and some medulla and is then fixed for light microscopy. Alternatively, the same sections may be taken for electron microscopy and the core is then divided longitudinally and their respective halves of the biopsies used for light microscopy and immunofluorescent studies, respectively. The division of the biopsy may be carried out within the gauze-containing Petri dish. Some workers section the needle core in a small longitudinal trough which has been fashioned from beeswax.

The single needle core obviously limits the amount of tissue available for each technique for examination. One further disadvantage seen more frequently with biopsies taken from shrunken kidneys is that the outer cortical piece selected for electron microscopy often contains glomeruli in advanced stages of sclerosis and is noncontributory. If sufficient time is available a second small section from the inner cortex will often overcome this problem. With two adequate needle cores containing cortex and medulla, one biopsy may be used in its entirety for light microscopy while the second may be divided for immunofluorescent and electron microscopic examination. Additional tissue may be available for glomerular culture. The piece selected for immunofluorescence may be dealt with in a number of ways. Rapid attachment to a microtome chuck with polyethylene glycol mounting medium (e.g., Miles OCT compound — see list of suppliers in Appendix) followed by immersion in liquid nitrogen is often employed. If available, a slurry of isopentane and nitrogen gives somewhat better morphological preservation. This is prepared by cautiously adding liquid nitrogen to about 50 mℓ of isopentane contained in a widemouthed insulated vessel. Care should be taken to avoid splashing the skin with slurry during mixing. Nitrogen is added, with stirring, until the isopentane begins to solidify. The slurry then has a temperature of −160°C. A less satisfactory alternative is to freeze the tissue by placing it in contact with a metal vessel or block chilled with a mixture of dry ice (solid carbon dioxide) dissolved in ethanol.

If the specimen must be transported or stored before sectioning it may be wrapped in aluminium foil and frozen by one of the above methods. The frozen biopsy is then placed in a (cold) tube and stored or transported in liquid nitrogen or dry ice. The latter is the more convenient and safer transport medium. If these materials are not available, it is essential that the tissue be stored at or below −70°C as deterioration will occur at higher temperatures.

An alternative ammonium sulfate-ethylmaleimide transport medium was developed by Michel et al.[1] The authors claim that this medium will preserve the activity of tissue-fixed immunoglobulins for several days without the need for freezing. We have not tested this medium with renal biopsies, but the method appears promising and details are given below.

Because of autolysis, post-mortem renal tissue may present problems, particularly for electron microscopic and immunofluorescent studies. However, sections of high technical quality may be obtained for electron microscopy and basement membrane structures are sufficiently durable to provide adequate ultrastructural detail, often many hours after death. Cytoplasmic detail is often grossly distorted with poor preservation of subcellular organelles. It has recently been shown that protein deposits of immunoglobulin, complement components, and fibrin maintain their antigenicity for up to 15 hr post-mortem.[2] Thus useful information may be obtained from immunofluorescent examination of tissues obtained at autopsy.

## II. AMMONIUM SULFATE-ETHYLMALEIMIDE TRANSPORT MEDIUM[1]

Tissue for immunohistochemical studies may be placed in this medium for several days before further processing. This permits transport of the tissue through the post etc. After removal from this medium the tissue is washed three times in the buffer (without the ammonium sulfate — 10 min each wash) and then frozen by the usual method.

| | |
|---|---|
| Buffer | 2.5 mℓ of 1 *M* potassium citrate buffer pH 7.0<br>5 mℓ of 0.1 *M* magnesium sulfate<br>5 mℓ of 0.1 *M* N-ethyl maleimide<br>87.5 mℓ distilled water<br>Adjust pH to 7.0 with 1 *M* potassium hydroxide |
| Working solution | To 100 mℓ of buffer add 55 g of ammonium sulfate |

## REFERENCES

1. **Michel, B., Milner, Y., and David K.,** Preservation of tissue-fixed immunoglobulins in skin biopsies of patients with lupus erythaematosus and bullous diseases. Preliminary report, *J. Invest. Dermatol.*, 59, 449, 1973.
2. **Sheibani, K., Tubbs, R. R., Valenzuela, R., and Deodhar, S.,** Reliability of immunofluorescence of renal tissue obtained at autopsy, *Am. J. Clin. Pathol.*, 72, 222, 1979.

Chapter 2

# FIXATIVES AND FIXATION

**David E. Allen and John P. Dowling**

## TABLE OF CONTENTS



## I. INTRODUCTION

Correct fixation of the renal biopsy is of great importance as improper preservation presents a severe handicap to the pathologist. Further, the effects of poor fixation cannot be rectified by subsequent processing steps, so particular care should be taken over this initial stage. Many factors influence fixation including delays before the tissue is placed in the fixative fluid, its penetration rate, the time of fixation, and the subsequent storage conditions. These factors are important for both optical and electron microscopy though the superior resolving power of the latter instrument necessarily places greater demands on the quality of fixation. It is convenient to deal separately with fixation techniques for optical microscopy in this section; methods for electron microscopy are covered later. However, the following points apply to both disciplines.

Tissues should be fixed as promptly as possible after excision, even a few minutes delay will produce observable ultrastructural changes. The tissue blocks should be of such a thickness that the fixing fluid readily penetrates throughout the block in a short period of time. This time will vary with the fixative and also inversely with temperature. While low temperatures retard fixation, they also slow autolytic changes so that improved fixation may follow longer immersion in a fixative at a low temperature. Note though that freezing of tissue blocks near 0°C must be avoided as considerable ice-crystal artifact will be produced. In the case of multicomponent fixatives the penetration rates of the various components will differ and if the specimen blocks are large, deeper layers of the tissue may show adverse effects due to reaction with only parts of the fixation mixture. The volume of fixative employed should be 15 to 20 times that of the tissue to be fixed and the container used should be of such dimensions that the tissue is not bent or folded. After the appropriate time interval the fixed tissue should be rinsed in a suitable washing medium and processed as soon as possible.

## II. OPTICAL MICROSCOPY

### A. Routine Methods

Many workers use formalin solutions as fixatives for renal biopsies. Usually these are prepared from commercial formalin (37 to 40% formaldehyde) diluted with either saline or (preferably) with a buffer (pH approximately 7) until the formaldehyde concentration is of the order of 4%. These fixatives are readily available and they allow the majority of staining reactions to be carried out successfully. However, formaldehyde is a rather "soft" fixative for renal tissue and often results in defects such as fraying of the brush border of the epithelium. Better results are obtained with Duboscq-Brasil solution.

In this ethanol-acetic acid-formaldehyde-picric acid mixture,[1] the picric acid acts as a "hard" fixative, overcoming the disadvantages of formaldehyde used alone. The solution penetrates well and fixes small biopsies rapidly. Staining methods of the Mallory and Masson type are enhanced by this fixation method. We have used this fixative successfully for a number of years and the complete formula and method are given below. An advantage that Duboscq-Brasil solution shares with buffered formaldehyde is that sufficient tissue antigenicity is retained to permit demonstration of some antigens with immunoperoxidase methods following paraffin embedding.

If material originally preserved with formalin is to be used, we have found it advantageous to apply Duboscq-Brasil solution as a post-fixative. The post-fixation is carried out by treating the tissue with DuboscqBrasil solution for several hours prior to processing. Subsequent staining is considerably enhanced by this treatment.

A disadvantage of Duboscq-Brasil solution is that it may cause red cells to be lysed. If this is considered undesirable, it may be overcome by a short pre-fixation of 10 min in Corrosive Formol. However, subsequent removal of mercury precipitates will also be required (see below).

Meadows and Schoemaker[2] have recommended Corrosive Formol as a superior fixative for renal biopsies since fixation is very rapid (30 to 45 min) and excellent histological detail, particularly of nuclei, is achieved. The mercury content of this fixative also potentiates some of the special staining procedures applied to renal biopsies. However, mercuric chloride is expensive, poisonous, and corrosive and its use results in the deposition of reduction products within the tissue. These must be removed with iodine and thiosulfate prior to staining. Even after this treatment, tissues fixed in mercury containing fluids are resistant to staining with the silver methenamine procedure. This difficulty can be overcome by treating deparaffinized sections with ammonia in alcohol overnight,[3] but silver staining times are still long and this may lead to excessive nonspecific silver deposition. Also, the silver impregnation tends to fade with time. Mercury-containing fixatives are also unsuitable for histochemical and immunohistochemical purposes. Full details of a Corrosive Formol fixative are given at the end of this section. Muehrcke and Pirani[4] recommended Helly's fluid as a fixative for renal biopsies. However, this mercury-containing fixative would seem to have no advantage over the above method.

Although mercury and chromate fixatives are not recommended for general histological purposes, Helly's fluid has been suggested as the fixative of choice when it is desired to demonstrate juxtaglomerular granules. The method used by Pitcock and Hartroft[5] in their application of Bowie's stain is given below. A possible alternative to the use of Helly's fluid in this method is the Corrosive Formol mixture suggested by Meadows and Schoemaker.

Chambers et al.[6] have suggested that glutaraldehyde be used as a fixative for routine histopathology and reported increased staining intensity with many stains. Agodoa et al.[7] have used this dialdehyde for fixing renal biopsies. It would be convenient to use the same fixative for both optical and electron microscopy, but after testing electron microscopy grade glutaraldehyde from several sources we cannot recommend the method. This dialdehyde penetrates tissue slowly and without long fixation times tissue preservation was poor and staining weak. It is notable that Chambers et al. used glutaraldehyde purified with activated charcoal and employed fixation times of 24 hr or more.

## III. FIXATIVES FOR OPTICAL MICROSCOPY

### A. Formol Saline Solution

| | |
|---|---|
| 37 to 40% formaldehyde solution (formalin) | 100 mℓ |
| Sodium chloride | 8.5 g |
| Tap or distilled water | 900 mℓ |

### B. Neutral Buffered Formaldehyde Solution

| | |
|---|---|
| 37 to 40% formaldehyde solution | 100 mℓ |
| Water | 900 mℓ |
| Sodium dihydrogen phosphate.1 $H_2O$ | 4 g |
| Disodium hydrogen phosphate.anhydrous | 6.5 g |

Adequate fixation is achieved in 16 to 24 hr; longer times may make sectioning more difficult. Tissues should remain in the fixative until processing into paraffin or plastic as washing reverses the fixation effect. Solution 2 is preferred as unbuffered formalin mixtures may be acidic and cause deposits to form in the tissues. See also the Section VI on fixatives for electron nicroscopy where an alternative phosphate buffered formalin mixture is described.

### C. Duboscq-Brasil Solution

| | | |
|---|---|---|
| 80% ethanol | 150 mℓ | |
| 37 to 40% formaldehyde solution | 60 mℓ | |
| Picric acid | 1 g | Solution A |
| Glacial acetic acid | 15 mℓ | Solution B |

Solution A should be prepared freshly at least once monthly and the acetic acid added immediately before use (14 parts of A to 1 part B). This avoides chemical decomposition and results in better fixation. We cannot recommend storage of the complete fixative as is sometimes suggested.

The minimum fixation time for a renal biopsy core is 1 hr, 4 to 5 hr is optimal, and 18 hr should not be exceeded. After fixation the tissue is washed in several changes of 70% ethanol, preferably overnight. The tissue may remain in this solution until processing is possible. This washing step is particularly important if the tissue is being processed into plastic. *Note:* Solid picric acid is explosive when dry.

### D. Corrosive Formol

| | |
|---|---|
| Saturated mercuric chloride | 90 mℓ |
| 37 to 40% formaldehyde solution | 10 mℓ |

The mixture should be prepared shortly before use as it becomes cloudy on standing. Fixation time is 30 to 45 min. Longer times should be avoided as biopsies become brittle and difficult to section. After fixation, tissues should be washed and stored in 70% ethanol as for Duboscq-Brasil solution. Corrosive formol is poisonous and corrosive and must be used with care; containers must not be of metal or have metal caps. After sectioning, the deparaffinized sections are hydrated via the following iodine-thiosulfate sequence to remove the mercury:

| | |
|---|---|
| Instead of the usual 70% alcohol step substitute 0.5% iodine in 70% alcohol; rinse in water | 5 min |
| Rinse in 5% sodium thiosulfate; wash in running water | 5 min |

If both mercurial and nonmercurial fixed material are included in the preparations to be stained; the iodine-thiosulfate procedure is harmless to the latter.

A special washing procedure is required if silver impregnation methods are to be used. After hydrating as described above slides are treated with 2% ammonia (concentrated) in 96% alcohol overnight.[3] The silver methenamine procedure will then require 60 to 90 min at 60°C for impregnation.

### E. Helly's Fluid for Demonstration of Juxtaglomerular Granules[5]

| | |
|---|---|
| Distilled water | 100 mℓ |
| Potassium dichromate | 2.5 g |
| Sodium sulfate | 1.0 g |
| Mercuric chloride | 5.0 g |
| Add immediately before use 37 to 40% formaldehyde solution | 5.0 mℓ |

Thin slices of tissues are fixed for 48 hr and washed in running tap water for 24 hr before embedding in paraffin or plastic.

# IV. ELECTRON MICROSCOPY

Fixatives for electron microscopy (EM) require more careful formulation than the mixtures used for optical microscopy in order to preserve ultrastructure and prevent extensive extraction. In general, an EM fixative consists of the fixing agent in a suitable buffer to maintain a contant pH value. Various salts may also be added to balance the ionic concentration and osmolarity of the fixative so that extraction is minimized and tissue components neither swell nor shrink during fixation.

EM fixatives are usually buffered to a pH of 7.4 to 7.6 though for many tissues there is little evidence that the pH is critical within the range of 6.5 to 8.0. It is difficult to quantify the most suitable values for the osmolarity of the fixative since little is known of the internal osmotic pressure of living tissue. A practical procedure is to select a fixative of known effectiveness in similar studies and to make adjustments if swelling or shrinkage of the tissue is observed. The fixatives selected for inclusion here have been shown to be satisfactory in this respect.

Osmium tetroxide is the best of the light microscope fixatives for preserving fine structure and it formed the basis of the earliest fixatives for EM. Sabatini et al.[8] later demonstrated the value of aldehydes as fixatives for EM and in particular the suitability of glutaraldehyde. This dialdehyde gives excellent preservation of a wide range of plant and animal tissues when followed by a second fixation in osmium tetroxide. This double fixation procedure had the advantage that specimens can be stored in buffer for considerable periods of time before further processing. A further advantage is that the fixative may be transported to and used in the biopsy room without undue risk. The toxicity and volatility of osmium tetroxide precludes its use in this manner. The convenience of this double fixation procedure coupled with the good ultrastructural preservation obtained has made it a standard procedure in most laboratories. Formaldehyde, freshly prepared from paraformaldehyde, compares favorably with glutaraldehyde and has the advantage of more rapid penetration into the specimen. Subsequently, mixtures of paraformaldehyde and glutaraldehyde[9] have proved to be superior to either aldehyde used alone for many specimens.

Osmium tetroxide is almost univerasally used as a secondary fixation step following primary aldehyde fixation. With fresh tissue the penetration rate of osmium tetroxide is very low and poor fixation in the center of tissue blocks can occur. The primary aldehyde fixation stabilizes the tissue sufficiently well to overcome these penetration artifacts and also the rate of penetration is increased over that of fresh tissue. A considerable amount of osmium is bound to the tissue following post-fixation. This osmium is bound in the form of "osmium blacks" which are amorphous electron opaque compounds of osmium. These reactions result in blackening of the tissue during post-fixation and also impart some electron opacity to the tissue. This staining effect is not ussually sufficient to enable examination of the tissue without further staining.

A number of buffers have been suggested for the control of pH in fixatives. Phosphate buffers are nontoxic and can produce excellent results. However, they do become slowly contaminated with microorganisms and they are prone to the formation of precipitates during fixation. This is presumably due to the formation of insoluble phosphates and may account for the sectioning difficulties and increased background granularity reported by some workers following the use of phosphate buffers. A number of formulas for the preparation of phosphate buffers are available but, providing they are of the same osmolarity, they give very similar results. Most of the formulas are based on that of Sorensen[22] and details for the preparation of this buffer are given below.

Cacodylate buffers were proposed for EM by Sabatini et al.[8] They are easy to prepare, stable indefinitely, and do not support the growth of microorganisms. In addition, the low concentrations of calcium ions added to fixatives to stabilize phospholipids do not result in precipitation. Sections from tissue fixed in the presence of cacodylate have greater inherent contrast in the electron microscope than do sections from similar material fixed in a phosphate buffered mixture. This effect is probably due to the binding of arsenic by tissue components, a factor which may have relevance to cytochemical studies. The disadvantage of cacodylates is that, because of their arsenic content, they are toxic. Recent reports[10] have stressed the dangers of this toxicity, and cacodylate buffers should be handled carefully in a fume cupboard and all skin contact should be avoided.

Other buffers chosen for use in electron microscopy have included veronal-acetate and s-collidine (ϒ-collidine or 2,4,6-trimethylpyridine). In fact veronal-acetate is a poor buffer system in the region of pH 5.2 to 7.5 and it also reacts with aldehydes to produce a substance with no buffering capacity in the physiological pH range.[11] Veronal buffers are highly toxic and must be used and disposed of with great care, they also support the growth of microorganisms. Their use cannot be recommended unless no alternative is available. Collidine is a good buffer in the region of pH 7.4 when half-neutralized with a strong acid and the buffer is stable indefinitely at room temperature. However, this buffer does cause considerable extraction of tissue components during fixation. Collidine is toxic, has a nauseating smell, and must be handled with extreme care. In consequence, this buffer system cannot be recommended for routine use.

Recently, excellent results have been reported following the use of PIPES (1,4-piperazine diethane sulfonic acid) buffer as the fixative vehicle for EM.[12,13] PIPES is not excessively toxic, does not precipitate common ions, and is a very effective buffer over the physiological pH range. Published micrographs show ultrastructural preservation equal to the best obtained with cacodylate or phosphate buffers. PIPES is especially recommended when long fixation times are unavoidable as it results in little extraction of tissue components and a freedom from the granular deposits sometimes found after prolonged fixation in other buffer systems. If PIPES is not available, we regard cacodylate buffer as the most suitable, although adequate precautions to protect workers against absorbtion of arsenic must be taken. If this cannot be ensured, phosphate buffers should be used.

Osmium tetroxide post-fixatives usually consist of a 1 or 2% solution of the oxide dissolved in a buffer. Frequently, the buffer used for the primary fixation is employed. Osmium tetroxide reacts only very slowly with cacodylate and phosphate buffers, but with PIPES buffer the fixative mixture darkens after approximately 1 hr at room temperature. This reaction does not appear to produce any adverse effects on the tissue and the extent of the reaction varies with the batch of material in use. Salemo and Brandao[12] have suggested that only a small proportion of the osmium tetroxide in solution is involved in the reaction. It is possible that the increased electron opacity of biopsies fixed in the presence of PIPES may be partly attributable to this reaction in a manner analogous to the use of phenylenediamine as a block stain[14] (see also Chapter 4). Dalton's chromate buffered osmium tetroxide[15] is recommended as a post-fixative. Chromate is a strong buffering agent and the solution is stable for at least 1 month at 4°C, enabling it to be kept as a stock solution. It is usually more economical to use this than to prepare small amounts of osmium fixatives each time tissue is processed. Dalton's fixative does not precipitate uranium salts (see below). A further advantage is that the strong yellow color of the fixative is a good guide to the efficiency of washing procedures. It is advisable to use all osmium fixatives at 4°C or at least at temperatures below 20°C to prevent the deposition of osmium reduction products throughout the tissue (see Figure 7 in Chapter 4).

The treatment of renal biopsies with uranyl acetate following post-fixation and before dehydration results in improved preservation of ultrastructure. This third fixation also results in a staining effect which gives improved contrast in the electron microscope. Uranyl acetate is particularly effective in the fixation of membranes as a consequence of the stabilization of phospholipids[16-18] although some other components (e.g., glycogen) may be extracted.[19] The fixative consists of 0.25 to 2.0% uranyl acetate in saline. Most fixation buffers (but not Dalton's) will precipitate insoluable uranium salts from solutions of uranyl acetate and tissue should be thoroughly washed with saline before treatment with the uranium salt. The fixative should be prepared at weekly intervals and stored at room temperature in the dark. Mixtures in which a precipitate has formed should be discarded. The staining effects of uranyl acetate are described in a later chapter.

Although producing excellent results, the above triple fixation sequence may be criticized on grounds of cost and time. In particular, the increased use of EM as a diagnostic aid in surgical and autopsy pathology has resulted in situations where there is demand for economical and short processing schedules and less emphasis on producing results of the highest quality. Several assessments of the value of formalin mixtures as primary fixatives have been made.[20] Formalin is generally readily available in clinical situations, dilute formalin mixtures keep well, and they are inexpensive. Early workers noted extreme variability in the quality of preservation following the use of formalin mixtures. This was probably due to the varying acidity and concentration of methanol which occurs in commercial formalin. However, a carefully buffered formaldehyde fixative prepared from a good grade of formalin can provide an adequate fixative. Carson et al.[21] tested various formalin mixtures and recommended a diluted formalin solution buffered with sodium dihydrogen phosphate and sodium hydroxide. This fixative is readily made in large quantities and produces results which are certainly adequate for diagnostic interpretation of a renal biopsy (Figure 5 in Chapter 4). Full details for preparing this mixture are given below. This fixative may also be used for optical microscopy though the results are less satisfactory than those obtained after fixation with Duboscq-Brasil solution.

If urgent electron microscopic examination of biopsy material is required a compressed fixation schedule may be followed. Only small pieces of tissue should be processed in this manner as some loss of ultrastructural detail may occur though preservation should be adequate for diagnosis. A suitable short processing schedule which may be adapted to use any of the above fixatives is given at the end of this section.

## V. APPENDIX FOR FIXATION (EM)

### A. Preparation of Buffers

#### *1. Sorensen's Phosphate Buffer*[22]

1. Prepare a 0.2 *M* solution of disodium hydrogen phosphate with: $Na_2HPO_4$ anhyd. (28.39 g), or $Na_2HPQ_4 \cdot 2H_2O$ (35.61 g), or $Na_2HPO_4 \cdot 7H_2O$ (53.65 g), or $Na_2HPO_4 \cdot 12H_2O$ (71.64 g) and distilled water to make 1000 mℓ.
2. Prepare a 0.2 *M* solution of sodium dihydrogen phospate with: $NaH_2PO_4 \cdot H_2O$ (27.6 g) or $NaH_2PO_4 \cdot 2H_2O$ (31.21 g) and distilled water to make 1000 mℓ.
3. Prepare a 0.2 *M* buffer by mixing x mℓ of 0.2 *M* disodium hydrogen phosphate with y mℓ of 0.2 *M* sodium dihydrogen phosphate.

| pH at 25°C | x mℓ | y mℓ |
|---|---|---|
| 6.8 | 24.5 | 25.5 |
| 7.0 | 30.5 | 19.5 |
| 7.2 | 36.0 | 14.0 |
| 7.4 | 40.5 | 9.5 |
| 7.6 | 43.5 | 6.5 |

*2. Cacodylate Buffer (0.2 M)*

Dissolve 21.4 g of sodium cacodylate in approximately 400 mℓ of distilled water. Adjust the pH of this solution to the value required with 0.2 *M* hydrochloric acid and then make up to 500 mℓ with more distilled water. *Warning:* Cacodylates should be treated as dangerously toxic chemicals. Take particular care to avoid inhalation or contact with the solid. Avoid all skin contact with the buffer as poisoning by skin absorbtion can occur.

*3. PIPES Buffer [Piperazine N-N′-bis(2 Ethane Sulfonic Acid)(0.2 M]*

Prepare a PIPES solution by disolving 34.24 g of the acid in approximately 400 mℓ of distilled water. Adjust to pH required with 0.2 *M* sodium hydroxide and make up to 500 mℓ with more distilled water.

*4. Dalton's Chromate Buffer*[15]

1. To 80 mℓ of a 5% solution of potassium dichromate add 2.5 *M* potassium hydroxide until the pH is 7.2
2. Add distilled water to make the final volume 100 mℓ.

This buffer is for Dalton's osmium tetroxide fixative (see below); it is not suitable for aldehyde fixatives.

**B. EM Fixatives**

*1. Glutaraldehyde-Formaldehyde Fixatives*

Commercial samples of glutaraldehyde can vary considerably in quality. For EM, samples of the aldehyde, usually supplied as a solution in water, should be clear and colorless and further dilution with water should not produce a precipitate. A number of manufacturers now supply an EM grade of glutaraldehyde, some of these are listed in the index of suppliers. On standing, solutions of glutaraldehyde undergo polymerization; for ordinary fixation purposes this is of little significance, but where the preservation of enzyme activity is of importance the presence of polymers may be deleterious. Pure glutaraldehyde has a single UV absorbance at 280 nm while the polymeric species absorb at 235 nm. For enzyme cytochemistry a sample of aldehyde having low absorbance at 235 nm should be used.

**Preparation of glut-formaldehyde fixative using a 70% (or 25%) aqueous solution of glutaraldehyde** — To 35 mℓ (50 mℓ) of the chosen buffer (0.2 *M* cacodylate, phosphate or PIPES pH 7.4) add 1.4 g (2.0 g) of paraformaldehyde. Warm gently, while shaking, to just below the boiling point. The paraformaldehyde should dissolve to give a clear solution. (Some samples of paraformaldehyde dissolve only with difficulty; in these cases addition of a few drops of 2.0 *M* sodium hydroxide should achieve solution). Cool the solution rapidly and then add the contents of a 2.0 mℓ ampule of 70% glutaraldehyde (Ladd) (or 8.0 mℓ of 25% solution). Rinse the ampule with a little distilled water adding the washings to the fixative. Add 0.14 mℓ (0.2 mℓ) of a 1.0 *M* solution of calcium chloride. Check the pH of the mixture and adjust if necessary to 7.4 by the dropwise addition of 2.0 *M* sodium hydroxide or hydrochloric acid. Bring the final volume to 70 mℓ (100mℓ) with distilled water. This fixative contains 2% formaldehyde and 2% glutaraldehyde. It is recommended that the fixative be used as fresh as possible but we have found little deterioration after storage at 4°C for 1 week.

**Preparation of glutaraldehyde fixative from 8% aqueous glutaraldehyde** — An adequate glutaraldehyde fixative may be rapidly prepared by diluting an 8% glutaraldehyde solution (Polysciences) with an equal volume of 0.2 *M* buffer.

*2. Formaldehyde (Formalin) Fixative*[21]

Formalin solution (37 to 40% formaldehyde), 10 mℓ
Sodium dihydrogen phosphate (anhyd), 1.86 g
Sodium hydroxide, 0.42 g
Distilled water to, 100 mℓ

*3. Osmium Tetroxide Fixatives*

**Preparation of a stock solution of osmium tetroxide** — Thoroughly clean a 1 g ampule of the tetroxide by washing in distilled water. All traces of the labels should be removed. Break open the ampule under 50 mℓ of water in a glass stoppered, dark glass bottle. The solid tetroxide will slowly dissolve to give a 2% solution. Solution may be hastened by shaking or, better, by placing the bottle in an ultrasonic bath. Warming the contents will also aid solution, but this must be done with care as the solid has a low melting point (40.6°C) and the material is dangerously volatile. This solution may be kept for several months in a tightly stoppered bottle at 4°C. It is advisable to keep the bottle of osmium tetroxide solution inside a closed container, e.g., a tin or jar. Any osmium vapor escaping from the stock bottle will rapidly blacken the surfaces of refrigerators or other storage compartments.

*Warning:* All contact with osmium tetroxide must be avoided; the material is caustic and rapidly blackens skin. The solid is toxic and has a high vapor pressure. The vapor is very dangerous to the eyes and mucous membranes. All handling of the solid and its solutions should be done in an efficient fume cupboard. Accidental spills of osmium tetroxide onto skin or clothing should be washed off immediately with large volumes of cold water, taking great care to avoid inhalation of the fumes. Spills on benches or apparatus should be treated immediately by mixing with excess 2 *M* sodium hydroxide solution. This converts the osmium to soluble and nonvolatile osmate. The strongly alkaline mixture should then be mopped up or flushed away with plenty of cold water.

**Preparation of an osmium fixative solution** — Equal volumes of 2% osmium tetroxide and the buffer of choice (0.2 *M* cacodylate, phosphate, or PIPES pH 7.4) are mixed. Providing that the buffer was carefully prepared, it is not necessary to check the pH of the fixative. The fixative mixture should be prepared shortly before use and only in quantities immediately required.

**Preparation of Dalton's chrome-osmium fixative** — Add 10 mℓ of 2% osmium tetroxide solution and 5mℓ of 3.4% aqueous sodium chloride to 5mℓ of chromate buffer (pH 7.2). There is no need to check the pH of the mixture which keeps for some months at 4°C. This fixative may be prepared as a stock solution for use as required.

*4. Uranyl Acetate Fixative*

Dissolve 1 g of uranyl acetate in 100 mℓ of saline solution (0.9% sodium chloride).

### C. Recommended Fixation Schedule for EM

1. Fix the selected portions of the biopsy for 2 to 3 hr. (or longer) at 4°C (refrigerator temperature), using the desired aldehyde fixative.
2. Wash several times (or overnight) in the fixation buffer or in saline.
3. Postfix in 1% osmium tetroxide in buffer or use Daltons fixative for 1 to 2 hr. at 4°C.
4. Wash several times in buffer or saline.
5. Fix/stain blocks in 1% uranyl acetate in saline for 30 to 60 min.
6. Wash several times in saline.

The tissue is now fixed and ready for processing into epoxy resin. Fixed tissue may be stored in saline at 4°C until further processing is possible.

**D. Compressed Schedule for Rapid Processing**

1. Fix pieces of tissue not larger than 0.5 mm in one dimension in a glutaraldehyde-formaldehyde fixative for 15 min at 4°C.
2. Rinse three times in the fixation buffer.
3. Postfix in buffered 1% osmium tetroxide or Daltons fixative for 15 min at 4°C.
4. Rinse two times in the fixation buffer.
5. Fix/stain with 2% uranyl acetate in saline for 15 min.

The tissue is now ready for dehydration and embedding with a rapid schedule (see Chapter 4, Section IV, A.1).

**E. Reclamation of Osmium Tetroxide**

Osmium is a rare and expensive element and very little of the osmium content of fixative solutions is incorporated into the tissue during fixation. Thus, if used fixative solutions are discarded most of the osmium is wasted. In order to prevent this and on grounds of economy it is desirable that the osmium be reclaimed from used fixatives. This is possible by the following techniques.

*1. Method of Kiernan*[23]

This method has been applied only to osmium solutions containing buffers (phosphate, cacodylate, barbiturate, collidine) and commonly used inorganic salts. For other mixtures see below. **All procedures must be carried out in an efficient fume cupboard.**

Old and used aqueous solutions of osmium tetroxide are collected in a large glass bottle with a tightly fitting screw cap. To 50 mℓ of these residues contained in a 1-ℓ flask add 5 mℓ concentrated sulfuric acid and 200 mℓ of 6% aqueous potassium permanganate. Mix well, cover the flask, and allow to stand for 30 min. If necessary, add more permanganate until a purple color persists in the mixture. Extract the mixture three times with 150 mℓ portions of carbon tetrachloride. Collect the organic layers and add to them 10 mℓ of absolute alcohol. Cover and leave for 48 hr to allow the osmium to precipitate as the dioxide. At the end of this time decant the colorless supernatant, add a further 10 mℓ of alcohol and again allow to stand for 24 hr. If there is no further precipitation, the used carbon tetrachloride is discarded. If more oxide is formed, it is filtered off and the filtrate again treated with alcohol. This is repeated until all the osmium is precipitated. If the separated dioxide adheres to the walls of the flask, a small amount of acetone is added and the material is scraped from the container with a glass rod. The suspension of the dioxide in acetone is filtered and the collected solid washed with acetone. The filter is allowed to dry (acetone is highly inflammable), the final drying being carried out in a vacuum desiccator. Finally, the dry dioxide is stored in a tightly stoppered bottle. According to Kiernan about 5 g of dry osmium dioxide has been obtained from each liter of residues. Since the composition of residues will generally be unknown, it is impossible to determine how much osmium is not recovered by the above procedure.

It is convenient to convert the osmium dioxide to the tetroxide in the form of a 2% solution from which fixatives can be prepared directly. To do this, 1 g of the dioxide is placed in a clean bottle and 45 mℓ of distilled water added. After suspending the solid, 1 mℓ of hydrogen peroxide (30% is added — *do not pipet by mouth* — and the mixture is loosely covered and allowed to stand for 30 min in a refrigerator. A further 1 mℓ of peroxide is then added and the mixture left to stand for a further 30 min. Dissolution of the dioxide should then be complete. The mixture is made up to 50 mℓ with distilled water to give an approximately 2% solution of osmium tetroxide. Any excess peroxide is decomposed by the osmium to oxygen and water.

*2. Alternative Method*

This process was developed as it was found preferable to store used fixatives by adding them to excess 50% alcohol. This reduces the tetroxide to the dioxide and osmium blacks and avoids the storage of large quantities of the toxic and volatile tetroxide solution. This method has been used with fixatives prepared with organic (PIPES) and chromate buffers. *Because of the presence of organic moieties in the fixative residues, the initial oxidation reaction described below may be violent. Use of a fume cupboard with a protective screen is essential.*

To a volume of fixation residues not exceeding 200 mℓ slowly add ½ the volume of concentrated pitric acid. The latter portions of the acid should be added with particular care, especially when nitrous fumes are produced and the mixture becomes warm. The reaction is very exothermic and may become violent; thus a large flask should be used and the addition of acid must be carried out in a fume cupboard.

Allow the reaction to proceed to completion and the contents of the flask to cool. Add solid sodium bicarbonate to neutralize most of the excess acid and to expel the nitrous fumes, but do not make alkaline. Extract the mixture with three portions of carbon tetrachloride each of 50 mℓ. Pool the organic layers and dry over anhydrous sodium sulfate. After filtering off the drying agent, osmium dioxide is precipitated from the carbon tetrachloride solution as in the above method.

## REFERENCES


1. **Zugibe, F. T.,** *Diagnostic Histochemistry,* C. V. Mosby, St. Louis, 1970, 130.
2. **Meadows, R. and Schoemaker, H.,** Improved processing for renal biopsies for light microscopy, *J. Clin. Pathol.,* 23, 548, 1970.
3. **Jones, D. E.,** Nephrotic glomerulonephritis, *Am. J. Pathol.,* 33, 313, 1957.
4. **Muehrcke, R. and Pirani, C. L.,** *Renal Disease,* Balck, D. A. K., Ed., Blackwell, Oxford, 1962, 425.
5. **Pitcock, J. A. and Hartcroft, P. M.,** The juxtaglomerular cells in man and their relationship to the level of plasma sodium and to the zona glomerulosa of the adrenal cortex, *Am. J. Pathol.,* 34, 863, 1958.
6. **Chambers, R. W., Bowling, M. C., and Grumley, P. M.,** Glutaraldehyde fixation in routine histopathology, *Arch. Pathol.,* 85, 18, 1968.
7. **Agodoa, L. C. Y., Striker, G. E., and Chi, E.,** Glycol methacrylate embedding for renal biopsy specimens for light microscopy, *Am. J. Clin. Pathol.,* 64, 655, 1975.
8. **Sabatini, D. D., Bensch, K., and Barrnett, R. J.,** Cytochemistry and electron microscopy. The preservation of cellular ultrastructure and enzymic activity by aldehyde fixation, *J. Cell Biol.,* 17, 19, 1963.
9. **Karnovsky, M. J.,** A formaldehyde-glutaraldehyde fixative of high osmolarity for use in electron microscopy, *J. Cell Biol.,* 27, 137A, 1965.
10. **Weakley, B. S.,** How dangerous is sodium cacodylate?, *J. Microsc. (Oxford),* 109, 249, 1976.
11. **Holt, S. J. and Hicks, R. M.,** Use of veronal buffers in formalin fixatives, *Nature,* 191, 832, 1961.
12. **Salema, R. and Brandao, I.,** The use of PIPES buffer in the fixation of plant cells for electron microscopy, *J. Submicrosc. Cytol.,* 5, 79, 1973.
13. **Baur, P. S. and Stacey, T. R.,** The use of PIPES buffer in the fixation of mammalian and marine tissues for electron microscopy, *J. Microsc. (Oxford),* 109, 315, 1977.
14. **Ledingham, J. M. and Simpson, F. O.,** The use of p-phenylenediamine in the block to enhance osmium staining for electron microscopy, *Stain Technol.,* 47, 239, 1972.
15. **Dalton, A. J.,** A chrome-osmium fixative for electron microscopy, *Anat. Rec.,* 121, 281, 1955.
16. **Silva, M. T., Guerra, F. C., and Magalhaes, M. M.,** The fixative action of uranyl acetate in electron microscopy, *Experientia,* 24, 1074, 1968

17. **Hayat, M. E.,** Principles and techniques of electron microscopy, in *Biological Applications,* Vol. 1, Van Nostrand Reinhold, New York, 1970.
18. **Silva, M. T., Mota, J. M. S., Melo, J. V. C., and Guerra F. C.,** Uranyl salts as fixatives for electron microscopy. Study of the membrane ultrastructure and phospholipid loss in bacilli, *Biochim. Biophys. Acta,* 233, 513, 1971.
19. **Farquhar, M. G. and Palade, G. E.,** Cell junctions in amphibian skin, *J. Cell Biol.,* 26, 263, 1965.
20. **Ashworth, C.T. and Stembridge, V. A.,** Utility of formalin fixed surgical and autopsy specimens for electron microscopy, *Am. J. Clin. Pathol.,* 42, 466, 1964.
21. **Carson, F. L., James, H., and Lynn, J. A.,** Formalin fixation for electron microscopy, a re-evaluation, *Am. J. Clin, Pathol.,* 59, 365, 1972.
22. **Dawson, R. M. C., Elliott, D. C., Elliott, W. H., and Jones, K. M.,** *Data for Biochemical Research,* 2nd ed., Clarendon Press, Oxford, 1969.
23. **Kiernan, J. A.,** Recovery of osmium tetroxide from used fixative solutions, *J. Microsc.,* 113, 77, 1978.

Chapter 3

# OPTICAL HISTOTECHNIQUES

**David E. Allen and John P. Dowling**

## TABLE OF CONTENTS

## I. INTRODUCTION

Tissue sections stained with histological dyes still provide the main technological basis for interpretation of the renal biopsy. The other procedures described in this book will add further, often essential, information but the primary guide to the pathological state of the tissue will come from viewing stained preparations in the light microscope. In particular, the histological findings will guide the selection of material for EM and determine the need for other special methods, e.g., immunomethods. For these reasons, the preparation of good material for light microscopy is of the utmost importance.

In order to prepare sections of the biopsy the tissue must be embedded in a suitable medium. Traditionally, paraffin wax has served as the embedment and this material is still used in many laboratories. More recently plastic embedments developed for EM have been adapted to optical methods. The plastic embedments offer the advantage that sections in the thickness range 0.25 to 2μm are easily obtained and there is greater freedom from shrinkage distortion and other artifacts. Thin sections improve the resolution of tissue components attained in the microscope and many workers consider section thicknesses of 2μm or less to be essential for the interpretation of a renal biopsy.[1] Thin sections of less than 2μm can be obtained from paraffin blocks particularly if modern waxes containing synthetic additives are used. However, greater technical expertise and more time are required if sections of reproducible quality are to be obtained. The thin sectioning ability of plastic blocks is only obtained at some expense. The plastic monomers are more costly than the highest quality wax preparations and a microtome capable of operating with glass knives is required. The monomers are also toxic and allergenic and so must be used with greater care. Staining reactions in plastic sections are less intense, this being partly due to the lesser amount of tissue present in the thinner sections.

**Table 1**
**COMPARISON OF PARAFFIN AND PLASTIC EMBEDDING**

| Paraffin | Plastic |
|---|---|
| Rapid processing is possible and automated processing equipment may be already installed in many laboratories | A 24-hr processing schedule is ususally required to permit the polymerization reaction to occur overnight |
| Reliable sectioning at less than 4 μm is technically demanding but no special equipment is required | Sectioning in the range 0.25 to 2 μm is easy providing a microtome equipped with a glass knife holder is available |
| Sections stain easily with standard techniques | Sections do not stain as intensely as paraffin embedded tissue and some modifications to technique are required; if epoxy resins are used, the embedment must be removed prior to staining |
| Embedding is reversible; tissue may be re-embedded in plastic at a later date (e.g., for electron microscopy); immunolabeling methods can be applied to paraffin sections | Embedding is irreversible; plastic blocks can be sectioned directly for electron microscopy; immunolabeling methods are usually not applicable |
| Regents of reliable quality are readily available; they may be stored for long periods | Reagents can be of variable quality and require careful storage to avoid deterioration |

We still retain the paraffin technique for urgent biopsies since very short processing schedules may be used. Rapid processing is not possible with plastic embedments since they generally require overnight polymerization for satisfactory results. Rapid processing may be necessary for the diagnosis of transplant rejection and oliguric renal failure, particularly due to diffuse crescentic glomerulonephritis. For a more detailed comparison of plastic and paraffin embedding see Table 1.

A number of plastic embedments have been suggested as being suitable for light microscopy. These fall principally into two groups; methods using methacrylates and those using epoxy resins. (For a review see Reference 2.) Of the methacrylates, glycol methacrylate (hydroxyethyl methacrylate) has proved to be the most popular medium while Spurr's low viscosity resin is the most suitable epoxy embedment for light microscopy. However, because of their suspected toxicity, the Spurr's monomers may eventually be unobtainable. It is therefore noted that EPON or ARALDITE resins may be used as alternative epoxy embedments. Of these alternatives, EPON is to be preferred, as the highly cross-linked ARALDITE is less easily removed prior to staining sectioned material. Full instructions for the preparation of EPON and ARALDITE monomers are given in the section on electron microscopy. These can be used as replacements for Spurr's medium in the methods given below, although extra care should be taken to ensure thorough infiltration with the monomer mix. The relatively large pieces of tissue used for optical microscopy are not easily penetrated by these more viscous epoxy mixtures. Extra time can be allowed for infiltration, but this is not necessary if an efficient agitation system is used.

The choice between glycol methacrylate (GMA) and an epoxy embedment is affected by many factors. Both methods have their advantages and disadvantages, some of which are summarized in Table 2.

Reliability is of paramount importance in biopsy studies and we have experienced problems with batch to batch variations in the quality of GMA monomers. For this reason we select an epoxy medium, preferably Spurr's, as the plastic embedment of choice. Occasionally, we have also received batches of Spurr's resin which stained poorly. The reasons for this are obscure, but the effect may be due to hydration of the monomers, reflecting poor storage or transport conditions.

**Table 2**
**COMPARISON OF GMA AND EPOXY-RESIN EMBEDDING**

| GMA | Epoxy resins |
|---|---|
| Polymerization can be unreliable as it is affected by monomer quality; good quality monomers can be difficult to obtain; the reaction is also inhibited by atmospheric oxygen and fixative residues | Polymerization reaction is reliable; good quality monomers readily available but they require careful storage to prevent hydration; fixative residues in moderate amounts do not inhibit polymerization |
| Staining properties affected by monomer quality; with good monomers staining intensity is comparable to a paraffin section of equal thickness | Staining properties affected by monomer quality; intensity of most stains is less than that attained with paraffin sections |
| Sections very easily at 0.5 to 2 μm but the sections are prone to the formation of creases and folds | Sections well at 0.25 to 2 μm though less readily than GMA and more frequent change of knife is necessary; sections are robust and easily handled |
| No need to remove plastic prior to staining though staining of the embedment may occur with poor quality monomers | Plastic removal is necessary prior to staining |
| Secitons adhere well to clean glass slides | Gelatinized slides are advisable; old or improperly stored monomers appear to accelerate section loss |

Some workers have obtained excellent results with GMA embedments[3] and for completeness we have included details of a GMA procedure found to be simpler and more reliable than others tested. This method uses a monomer mixture consisting only of GMA and polyethylene glycol (PEG 400) and the catalyst is azobisisobutyronitrile. The PEG 400 and the catalyst are readily available in high purity and thus only the quality of the GMA need be checked. Also, azobisisobutyronitrile is more stable than the usual peroxide catalysts, it may safely be stored as a dry powder, and the polymerization reaction proceeds more smoothly.

## II. PARAFFIN EMBEDDING

A rapid dehydration, infiltration, and embedding sequence is described. This procedure gives good results and longer schedules offer no advantage, although they may be used if more convenient. For embedding, a modern wax preparation containing plasticizers is strongly recommended (e.g., Paraplast or Tissue-prep). Many tissue blocking systems are now available (e.g., Tissue-Tek) and any of these may be used.

Tissue from fixative (at least 2 hr fixation):

| | |
|---|---|
| 95% alcohol | Two changes 10 min each |
| Absolute alcohol | Two changes 20 min each |
| Xylene | Two changes 15 min each |
| Paraffin wax I | 10 min (in vacuo) |
| Paraffin wax II | 20 min (in vacuo) |
| Embed in fresh wax | |

Sections should be cut at a thickness of 1 to 2μm and for this a good quality microtome is essential. The actual type is immaterial, but the machine must be of robust construction and the advance mechanism in good order. The knife should be freshly sharpened and it is an advantage to cool both knife and block in the freezing compartment of a refrigerator before use. If dry ice is available, a few lumps of this material held in a sieve which is clamped above the knife and block will maintain these at a cool temperature. Under these conditions thin sections can be obtained more easily, but the markings on the advance mechanism of the microtome may not be reliable and initially section thickness should be checked by microscopy.

The sections are spread on a water bath (45°C) and picked up on clean glass slides. It is advantageous to sequentially number the slides (and hence determine the order of the sections). Frequently, pathological changes are localized in one or several sections of the biopsy and it is desirable to stain alternate sections so that much of the tissue specimen is examined.

The slides are then dried in an oven (70 to 80°C) before staining. Further details of paraffin histotechnique may be found in standard texts.[4] Details of staining reactions are given following Section III.

## III. PLASTIC EMBEDDING

### A. Glycol Methacrylate

Glycol methacrylate (GMA, hydroxyethyl methacrylate) is available from a number of sources, but it is important that only good quality material be purchased (see list of suppliers in the Appendix). It is best to specify methacrylate of low acid content as acidic impurities, principally derivatives of acrylic acid, may cause irregular polymerization. Even so, particular batches may polymerize poorly or not at all. In these cases a number of purification procedures are possible. The simplest procedure is to stir the GMA with activated charcoal.[5] Batches of 50 mℓ of the GMA are stirred with 2 g of charcoal for 1 hr. The mixture is filtered and the process repeated. This procedure will remove the inhibitor added to commercial GMA to prevent spontaneous polymerization, but has only slight effect upon acidic impurities. Once present, these are difficult to remove by any process except vacuum distillation. (Bp 50°C at 11 mm Hg.) An ion-exchange process has been recommended by Bennett et al.,[5] but we have found this to be time consuming and on a small scale the yield of purified methacrylate is poor. An alternative procedure is to shake the GMA with an equal volume of 2 *M* sodium hydroxide solution saturated with common salt. The organic layer is separated and the process repeated. The GMA is finally washed with saturated salt solution and then dried over anhydrous sodium sulfate. A small amount of residual salt has no effect upon polymerization. This procedure also results in some loss of GMA, but is simpler to carry out than the ion-exchange process. A simple test of the quality of the monomer is to dilute a sample with an equal quantity of water. Satisfactory samples of the monomer should not produce any precipitate or cloudiness under these conditions.

Infiltration and embedding of the fixed and washed tissue is carried out as follows. It is important that washing of the tissue be carried out as detailed in the fixation schedules since residual fixatives will inhibit polymerization.

Tissue from washing in 70% alcohol:

| | |
|---|---|
| 90% alcohol | 30 min |
| Absolute alcohol | 30 min |
| 50% GMA/alcohol | 15 min |
| 100% GMA | 15 min |
| Complete GMA mixture | 30 min |

Although GMA is water soluble, better infiltration is obtained after dehydration. The complete GMA mixture is as follows:

| | |
|---|---|
| GMA | 9.5 mℓ |
| PEG 400 | 0.5 mℓ |
| AZOBIS | 0.4 g |

Embed in gelatin capsules using fresh monomer. It is convenient to place the tissue in the capsule and then add the monomer mix from a disposable syringe, using the syringe needle to pierce a hole in the capsule. A second hole allows for the escape of air and excess monomer. It is important to completely fill the capsule as oxygen inhibits polymerization. Most renal biopsies can be accommodated in gelatin capsules, but if necessary other embedding molds may be used. Open molds (e.g., plastic or foil dishes) can be sealed with wax or covered with polythene film to exclude oxygen. If large numbers of blocks are being processed, they can be placed in a sealed container together with a lighted candle. Polymerization is carried out at 40°C. A simple wire frame can be constructed to support the capsules in the oven.

**B. Spurr's Epoxy-Resin**

A number of suppliers (see Appendix) market the components for this epoxy-resin system, both as separate reagents and also in the form of kits. There is some variation in the quality of chemicals from different sources and in general it is not a good idea to mix chemicals from different manufacturers. Poor adhesion of sections to slides and weak staining reactions are evidence of poor quality or hydrated mononers. We have found the Spurr's reagents supplied by Polysciences, Inc. (see Appendix) to be of a consistently high standard. The monomers should be carefully stored in a dry atmosphere to avoid hydration and the hardener (nonenylsuccinic anhydride, NSA) especially must be kept tightly capped. Refrigerator storage is not necessary. Unopened reagents have a long shelf-life.

The normal resin mixture recommended by Spurr[6] is suitable for renal biopsies and has the following composition:

| | |
|---|---|
| Vinylcyclohexane dioxide (VCA) | 5 g |
| DER 736 | 3 g |
| NSA | 13 g |
| S1 accelerator (dimethylaminoethanol) | 0.2 mℓ |

The first three components are carefully weighed out and well mixed. The accelerator is added from a 1.0-mℓ disposable syringe and again the components are thoroughly mixed. The complete mixture will keep for 1 day at room temperature and for 3 days at 4°C. If stored in a refrigerator, care must be taken to avoid condensation of moisture in the mixture.

Because of the toxicity of this resin mixture, gloves should be used during its use and care taken to avoid contact and inhalation of vapors. If resin is spilled on the skin, wash off with excess soapy cold water. Do **not** use organic solvents as these will speed the passage of the resin through the skin.

## IV. PROCESSING

Tissues from washing in 70% alcohol:

| | |
|---|---|
| 90% alcohol | 15 min |
| Absolute alcohol | 3 × 30 min |
| Xylene | 2 × 20 min |
| 50% xylene/50% resin | 30 min |
| 100% resin | 60 min |

Embed in fresh resin in a suitable mold and polymerize overnight at 70°C. Suitable molds are formed by plastic vial caps, aluminum foil dishes, and a variety of commercially available embedding molds (see EM section of Appendix).

We have found that sections of tissue embedded in Spurr's resin stain more intensely if the following additional steps are included in the dehydration/infiltration sequence. The reason for this is not known, but the heat and solvent effect of the wax may achieve enhancement in a similar manner to Lendrum's trichloroethylene "degreasing" treatment for enhancing the MSB method for fibrin (see Section V.B and Reference 11).

After clearing in xylene, transfer to paraffin wax (Paraplast, etc.) at 60°C for 2 × 20 min. Allow to cool and solidify for 30 min. Re-melt wax and remove tissues into xylene for 3 × 30 min. Continue infiltration with 50% resin/xylene as above.

Recently, machines designed to automatically process tissues into plastic embedments have been marketed (e.g., Sakura and Reichert Processors, see Appendix). Where a high volume of work is envisaged these would greatly reduce the staff work load.

### A. Sectioning of Plastic Embedded Tissue

Methacrylate and Spurr's blocks are generally sectioned with glass knives, although the former can be cut with a steel knife. If a steel knife is used, the sections are collected from the knife with a brush and floated out on a water bath. When sectioning with a glass knife the process is similar to that employed for electron microscopy (see Chapter 4, Section V). Indeed, an ultramicrotome which incorporates a coarse advance mechanism (0.5 to 2$\mu$m) may be used, although glass-knife holders are now available for many standard histology microtomes. In general, the coarse advance fitted to ultramicrotomes is manually operated, and it may be more convenient to use an ordinary microtome with auto-advance over the required range. Some manufacturers now produce microtomes especially designed for the sectioning of plastic embedded tissue (e.g., Sorvall JB 4) and these have improved facilities for trimming plastic blocks and greater maneuverability of the specimen and knife holder. If a large amount of plastic embedding is contemplated, purchase of such a unit would be worthwhile.

The sectioning of correctly polymerized plastic blocks with glass knives poses few problems. Methacrylate is perhaps the easier material to section as it is softer. However, it is also hydrophilic and careful trimming of the block face is necessary to avoid persistent wetting with water from the knife trough. The sides of the block should be steeply angled and surplus (empty) plastic minimized. Methacrylate sections are also prone to creasing and they do not easily form ribbons. It is usually best to cut one section at a time. Any creases may be gently teased out using forceps, a wire loop, or an eyelash attached to an orange stick. Alternatively, the sections may be spread with ammonia vapor by gently waving over them a triangle of filter paper soaked in aqueous ammonia. Dilute ammonia solution (10 to 15%) may also be used as the trough liquid although the fumes may be troublesome to the microtomist. The sections are transferred from the knife trough by picking up with a wire loop. They are then floated onto a drop of water on a clean microscope slide. If Spurr's resin is the embedment, it is advisable to use gelatin-coated slides to prevent section loss. The method for coating slides with gelatin is given below. Drying of the sections is conveniently accomplished on a 60°C hot plate.

The sectioning of Spurr's embedded material is performed in a similar manner. However, this resin is harder and more frequent knife changes will be necessary. It should be noted though that superficial scratches in sections of this material can be ignored as they will disappear when the plastic is removed prior to staining. Spurr's resin sections will form ribbons, but the length of a renal core biopsy may preclude the cutting of more than one section at a time. These sections are less prone to creasing, but if necessary they may be spread by exposure to chloroform vapor from a triangle of filter paper. Again, the sections are picked up with a wire loop and transferred to gelatin coated slides. Drying is carried out on the 60°C hot plate. Again, it is desirable that slides from the biopsy be numbered sequentially (see Section III).

### B. Gelatin Coating of Slides for Optical Microscopy

1. Ensure slides are chemically clean and grease-free by rinsing in detergent followed by thorough washing in water or, alternatively, treat slides with chromic acid and then wash thoroughly in water.
2. Bring slides to temperature in an oven at 50 to 60°C and then dip into 0.5% aqueous gelatin solution at 56°C. Drain, then immerse in 10% aqueous formalin held at 40°C.
3. Drain the slides and dry in a well ventialated oven at 50 to 60°C for 2 hr.

### C. Chromic Acid

This reagent is prepared as follows. To 500 g of sodium dichromate (commercial grade) dissolved in 1 ℓ of tap water and contained in a large pyrex glass flask, *slowly* add concentrated sulfuric acid. The acid is added at such a rate as to prevent boiling and with constant stirring. The addition is continued until crystals of chromic acid just begin to form in the solution (approximately 1 ℓ). *Note:* The above solution will become very hot during the addition of the acid. Extreme care should be taken during the addition to avoid splashing, eye protection is advised, and the reaction should be carried out under a fume hood. Chromic acid may explode if brought into contact with oxidizable materials and only clean glassware should be used in its preparation. Glassware to be cleaned must be rinsed free of organic solvents before treatment with chromic acid. The acid is extremely corrosive towards skin and clothing and will also slowly oxidize plastics such as polyethylene. Although an excellent cleaning agent, many laboratories caution against the use of this acid because of the hazards involved. It should never be prepared or used without adequate supervision and always treated with great respect.

## V. STAINING

Methods are given for both plastic and paraffin sections; where only one time is stated this is used for both types of sections. In the case of tissues embedded in Spurr's resin and paraffin, the embedment must be removed prior to staining. Sections of GMA embedded tissue may be stained immediately after drying without removal of the plastic.

### A. Removal of Spurr's Resin

1. Soak the slides for 10 to 30 min in either saturated sodium hydroxide in absolute ethanol* or saturated sodium methoxide in methanol.**

The time required depends on the condition of the solution. It is possible to see whether the plastic has been removed by rinsing the slide in absolute alcohol and examining the

* For this solution 99.7 to 100% ethanol should be used and not commercial "absolute alcohol". Elsewhere in this section the term "absolute ethanol" can be taken to mean a commercial grade ethanol or methylated spirit.

** This solution is prepared by cautiously adding *small* lumps of sodium metal to approximately 50 mℓ of anhydrous methanol. The metal dissolves with a brisk effervescence and hydrogen is evolved *(care flammable)*. Take care not to add the sodium at such a rate that the methanol boils. Continue to add the metal until the rate of dissolution is very slow. Dispose of any residual sodium with care as it reacts violently with water. These solutions should be stored in tightly capped containers as they are hygroscopic and the presence of water reduces their effectiveness.

section macroscopically. If plastic removal is complete, there will be no outline of embedding medium around the section. EPON or ARALDITE embedments require a longer reaction time than Spurr's resin.

Either of these solutions will readily dissolve the Spurr's embedment when fresh, but they gradually deteriorate with use and storage. The methoxide mixture has the stronger action and the better keeping qualities and it is more reliable. It is therefore recommended providing adequate care can be exercised in the handling of the sodium metal. The solutions should be changed when plastic removal becomes slow or subsequent staining is unsatisfactory.

2. Rinse the slide in absolute alcohol (2 changes)
3. Rinse the slide in 90% alchohol
4. Rinse the slide in 70% alchohol
5. Rinse the slide in 50% alchohol
6. Rinse the slide in water

### B. Removal of Paraffin Wax

Paraffin wax is removed from the sections by dissolution in xylene. The slides are then brought to water via graded alcohols as described above.

## VI. STAINING METHODS

### A. Hematoxylin and Eosin

*1. Technique*

| | Times | |
|---|---|---|
| | **Plastic** | **Paraffin** |
| 1. Bring sections to water | | |
| 2. Stain in hematoxylin (Harris's or preferably Carazzi's*) | 8 min | 4 min |
| 3. Rinse in water | | |
| 4. Differentiate briefly in acid alcohol (1%) hydrochloric acid in 70% alcohol—this step is not required if Carazzi's hematoxylin is used) | | |
| 5. Wash in water | | |
| 6. Blue in Scott's solution** | | |
| 7. Wash in water | | |
| 8. Stain in 2% aqueous eosin | 10 min | 4 min |
| 9. Rinse very briefly in absolute alcohol and transfer to xylene | | |
| 10. Rinse in fresh xylene and mount in synthetic medium | | |

*2. Results*

| | |
|---|---|
| Nuclei, cytoplasmic RNA, some calcium salts, urates, bacteria (weakly) | Blue |

* Carazzi's hematoxylin: hematoxylin, 1 g; sodium iodate, 0.2g; glycerol, 200 mℓ; potassium aluminum sulfate, 50 g; water to 1ℓ.

** Scott's tap water substitute: sodium bicarbonate, 3.5 g; magnesium sulfate, 20.0g; water to 1ℓ; add a crystal of thymol to prevent mold growth.

| | |
|---|---|
| Muscle, keratin, course elastic fibers, fibrin, fibrinoid | Bright red |
| Collagen, reticulin, nerve fibers, amyloid | Pink |
| Red blood cells | Orange |

## B. Periodic Acid-Schiff's (PAS) and Hematoxylin

### *1. Technique*

| | Time | |
|---|---|---|
| | **Plastic** | **Paraffin** |
| 1. Bring sections to water | | |
| 2. Oxidize in 1% periodic acid (aqueous) | 30 min | 10 min |
| 3. Wash in water and then rinse in distilled water | 10 min | 5 min |
| 4. Treat with Schiff's reagent* | 60 min | 15 min |
| 5. Wash in running water | 20 min | 10 min |
| 6. Stain in hematoxylin (Harris's or Carazzi's) | 8 min | 4 min |
| 7. Wash in water | | |
| 8. Differentiate briefly in 1% acid alcohol if required | | |
| 9. Wash in water | | |
| 10. Blue in Scott's solution | | |
| 11. Wash in water | | |
| 12. Dehydrate, clear, and mount (DCM) in synthetic resin | | |

In order to emphasize basement membrane structure, exposure to the Schiff's reagent is longer than usual.

### *2. Results*

| | |
|---|---|
| Nuclei | Blue or blue-black |
| Basement membranes and other PAS-positive material | Magenta |

## C. Silver Impregnation Method

### *1. Technique*

| | Time | |
|---|---|---|
| | **Plastic** | **Paraffin** |
| 1. Bring section to water | | |
| 2. Oxidize with 1% aqueous periodic acid | 30 min | 10 min |
| 3. Wash in water | | |
| 4. Rinse in distilled water | | |
| 5. Place section in a glass coplin jar fitted with a glass lid and containing | 30—50 min | 25—40 min |

* Schiff's reagent: Dissolve 1 g of basic fuchsin in 200 mℓ of boiling distilled water. Shake for 5 min and cool to exactly 50°C. Filter and add to the filtrate 20 mℓ of 1 *M* hydrochloric acid. Cool to 25°C and add 1 g of sodium or potassium metabisulfite. Stand this solution in the dark for 14 to 24 hr. The mixture should now have only a pale straw color; if it is still darkly colored, the fuchsin used is of poor quality and a fresh batch should be substituted. Add 2 g of activated charcoal and shake for 1 min. Filter. Keep the filtrate in the dark at 0 to 4°C. Allow to reach room temperature before use.

| | | |
|---|---|---|
| 50 mℓ of silver methanemine solution;* place the jar in a water bath at 60°C; check the section visually and/or microscopically at frequent intervals after 30 (25) min rinse in distilled water before and after handling; stop the reaction when basement membranes are adequately stained | | |
| 6. Rinse in distilled water | | |
| 7. Tone with 0.1% gold chloride | 1 min | 2—5 min |
| 8. Rinse in distilled water | | |
| 9. Treat with 5% sodium thiosulfate in water (if plastic sections tend to detach from the slide, this step may be omitted) | 5 min | 2 min |
| 10. Counterstain with the desired method | | |

*2. Results*

| | |
|---|---|
| Basement membranes | Black |
| Other tissue features dependent on the chosen counterstain | |

If the biopsy was fixed in the presence of mercuric chloride, mercury precipitate should be removed with iodine and thiosulfate and the sections treated with ammonia and alcohol overnight (see Chapter 2). The silver impregnation may fade with time after this form of processing. This effect may be reduced by omitting the toning step (Step 7).

Counterstains used after the silver methenamine are as follows.

## D. Masson Trichrome

*1. Technique*

| | Time | |
|---|---|---|
| | **Plastic** | **Paraffin** |
| 1. Bring sections to water | | |
| 2. Stain with Weigert's iron hematoxylin until nuclei are adequately stained; differentiated and blue; wash in water | | |
| 3. Stain in the red mixture** | 30 min | 3—5 min |
| 4. Wash in water and with paraffin sections differentiate with 1% aqueous phosphotungstic acid until the connective tissue is almost unstained; wash again in water | | 5—15 min |
| 5. Drain slide and stain in 2% light green in 2% acetic acid | 2—3 min | 2—3 min |

* Silver methenamine solution: Stock solution — 100 mℓ of 3% aqueous hexamine (hexamethylenetetramine) with 5 mℓ of 5% silver nitrate solution. Working solution — 25 mℓ stock solution is added to 25 mℓ of distilled water and 2 mℓ of 5% aqueous borax is added. All glassware used for the silver solution must be chemically clean and only glass distilled water should be used. Failure to observe these precautions may result in considerable random silver deposition. Silver deposits may be removed from glassware by rinsing with dilute (10%) nitric acid.

** Red mixture: 6 mℓ 1% Ponceau 2R, 2 mℓ 1% acid fuchsin, 1 mℓ 1% azophloxine, 9 mℓ 2% acetic acid, and water to 100 mℓ.

6. Blot the slide dry, rinse in xylene, and mount in synthetic medium

In the case of plastic sections the action of the acidified light green solution is critical as it serves both to differentiate the red mixture and also acts as the connective tissue stain. The green dye should be applied until the red is just displaced from connective tissue present in the section. If difficulty is experienced in this step, a fresh light green solution should be prepared.

*2. Results*

| | |
|---|---|
| Nuclei | Blue-black |
| Muscle, red blood cells, fibrin | Red |
| Connective tissue | Green |

**E. Chromotrope 2R**

*1. Technique*

1. Bring sections to water
2. Stain with 2% chromotrope 2R in 0.02 *M* hydrochloric acid for 1 hr (paraffin and plastic sections)
3. Blot the slide dry, rinse in xylene, and mount in synthetic medium

*2. Results*

| | |
|---|---|
| Nuclei and cytoplasm | Pink |
| Proteinaceous deposits | Red |

**F. Chromotrope-Aniline Blue**

*1. Technique*

1. Stain as above up to and including Step 2
2. Wash off the chromotrope 2R with 0.5% aniline blue in 0.02 *M* hydrochloric acid; leave this stain on the sections for 2 min
3. Rinse very briefly in water
4. Blot the slide dry, rinse in xylene, and mount in synthetic medium

*2. Results*

As for Chromotrope 2R but connective tissue stains blue.

The hematoxylin-eosin stain may also be used as a counterstain to the silver methenamine method.

**G. Alternative Method for Glomerular Protein Deposits**

This procedure was recommended by Gamble[7] who describes the procedure as easily reproducible. Proteinaceous deposits are selectively stained a deep blue and contrast sharply with adjacent glomerular structures. The author claims excellent correlation with immunofluorescent and EM studies and suggests that the stain enables characterization of a large variety of glomerular lesions by light microscopy alone.

*1. Solutions*

Stock Schiff's reagent

| | |
|---|---|
| Stock light green | |
| Light green SF yellowish (CI 670) | 0.2 g |
| Distilled water | 100 mℓ |
| Acetic acid | 0.2 mℓ |

Working strength light green
Add 10 mℓ of stock to 40 mℓ of distilled water; the pH should be 3.6

Gamble recommended fixation in Helly's fluid for 30 min to 1 hr followed by post-fixation in 10% buffered formalin for at least 2 hr. Before the post-fixation step the tissue is washed for 1 hr in running water. We prefer the Duboscq-Brasil fixative which avoids both the post-fixation step and also removal of the mercury precipitate.

### *2. Method*

1. Bring sections to water; if fixed in Helly's fluid, remove the mercury precipitate by the following steps, otherwise proceed to Step 2

| | | |
|---|---|---|
| Treat with Lugol's iodine | 7 | min |
| Wash in water | 6 | min |
| Treat with 5% sodium thiosulfate | 3 | min |
| Wash in water | 6 | min |
| 2. Oxidize in 0.5% periodic acid | 5 | min |
| 3. Wash in water | 6 | min |
| 4. Treat with Schiff's reagent | 15 | min |
| 5. Wash in running water | 10 | min |

6. Dip the slides one at a time in 0.05% light green solution until the sections turn green (40 to 50 dips)
7. Differentiate in 95% alcohol until pale blue-green (4 to 5 dips)
8. Dehydrate in 95% alcohol and in 2 changes of absolute alcohol; check the slides microscopically; background should be pale blue-green; if too green take back to water to remove the excess or if too weak re-stain in the light green mixture
9. When differentiation is correct dehydrate in a final change of absolute alcohol, clear in xylene, and mount in synthetic medium.

### *3. Results*

| | |
|---|---|
| Glomerular immune complexes | Deep blue |
| Basement membranes | Magenta |
| Mesangial matrix | Magenta |
| Cytoplasm and nuclei | Pale blue-green |
| Tubular reabsorption droplets | Deep blue |
| Tubular casts | Blue-green to reddish-blue depending on aldehyde content |
| Fibrin | Deep blue |
| Hyaline | Deep blue to red blue |
| Amyloid | Light magenta to bluish red |

## H. Weigert's Elastic Fiber Technique[8]

### *1. Solutions*

| | |
|---|---|
| Acidified potassium permanganate solution | |
| 0.25% aqueous potassium permanganate | 47.5 mℓ |
| 3% aqueous sulfuric acid | 2.5 mℓ |
| These are conveniently kept as stock solutions and mixed shortly before use. | |
| | |
| Oxalic acid solution | 2 g |
| 5% aqueous oxalic acid | |
| | |
| Weigert's resorcinol fuchsin solution | |
| Basic fuchsin | |
| Resorcin | 4 g |
| Distilled Water | 200 mℓ |

| | |
|---|---|
| 30% aqueous anhydrous ferric chloride | 25 mℓ |
| 95% alcohol | 4 mℓ |
| concentrated hydrochloric acid | |

Dissolve the basic fuchsin and the resorcin in the distilled water, bringing to a boil in a porcelain evaporating dish. While still boiling, slowly add the ferric choloride solution with continuous stirring. Continue this boiling and stirring for approximately 5 min. Cool and filter into a conical flask taking care that all the available precipitate is collected. Discard the filtrate. Now dry the flask and put into it the filter paper containing the precipitate. Add the alcohol and heat gently on a hot plate until the precipitate is dissolved. Remove the filter paper, add the concentrated hydrochloric acid, cool, and filter. Make up the final volume to 200 mℓ by pouring fresh 95% alcohol through the filter paper. Note that the purified fuschins recommended for Schiff's reagent commonly gives inferior results. This procedure is based on that given by Cook.

### *2. Technique*

1. Take sections to water
2. Treat with the acidified permanganate solution for 5 min; wash and bleach with oxalic acid for approximately 1 min
3. Wash well in water and rinse in absolute alcohol
4. Stain in the elastin solution; the time will vary with the batch of the solution but typically requires 1 to 3 hr at room temperature
5. Wash in water and differentiate in acid alcohol until the background is clear of stain; wash well in water
6. Counterstain as desired, e.g., neutral red, eosin, or van Gieson
7. Dehydrate, clear, and mount

### *3. Results*

| | |
|---|---|
| Elastic fibers | Dark blue-black |
| Background | Dependent on counterstain used |

## I. Gomori's Elastic Method[8]

### *1. Solutions*

| | |
|---|---|
| Acidified permanganate and oxalic acid | See above |

Aldehyde fuchsin
Dissolve 1 g of basic fuchsin in 100 mℓ of 60% alcohol.
Add concentrated hydrochloric acid (1 mℓ) and paraldehyde (2 mℓ).
Allow to blue at room temperature for at least 2 days before use. Store at 4°C. The solution should keep for 1 to 3 months. Deterioration will produce increased backgound staining.

### *2. Technique*

1. Take sections to water
2. Treat with the acid permanganate solution for 1 min; wash, bleach with the oxalic acid solution, then wash well in water
3. Rinse in 70% alcohol.
4. Stain with the aldehyde fuchsin solution for 4 min
5. Rinse well in 70% alcohol, then in water
6. Counterstain, e.g., with 0.1% aqueous methylene blue or 0.2% light green in 0.2% acetic acid
7. Dehydrate, clear, and mount

### *3. Results*

| | |
|---|---|
| Elastin and sulfated mucins | Purple |
| Background | Dependent on counterstain used |

## J. Martius Scarlet Blue Method[2]

### *1. Solutions*

Staining solution: stock solutions

A. 0.1% martius yellow (naphthol yellow) in 95% alcohol containing 2% phosphotungstic acid
B. 1% brilliant crystal scarlet R in 2.5% acetic acid
C. 0.5% aniline blue in 1% acetic acid

Working solution

| | |
|---|---|
| Solution A | 1 part |
| Solution B | 3 parts |
| Solution C | 2 parts |

### *2. Technique*

Good results are obtained following fixation with mercury-containing fixatives or glutaraldehyde. Duboscq-Brasil fixation has produced inconsistent staining with this trichrome in our hands. Sections may be mordanted in aqueous mercuric chloride. After treatment with mercuric chloride, mercury deposits must be removed with an iodine/thiosulphate sequence. If these materials are not available, sections can be treated with trichloroethylene for 24 hr after removing the embedment.[9]

1. Stain nuclei with Weigert's iron hematoxylin — 10 min
2. Differentiate in 1% acid alcohol and wash in water
3. Stain in the working MSB solution — 10 min
4. Rinse in water then dehydrate, clear, and mount.

### *3. Results*

| | |
|---|---|
| Fibrin | Red |
| Muscle | Pale red |
| Nuclei | Blue-black |
| Collagen | Blue |
| Red blood cells | Yellow |

## K. Congo Red Method for Amyloid[8]

There is some evidence that overlong exposure of plastic sections to either sodium hydroxide or sodium methoxide solutions can result in the extraction of amyloid. For this reason when staining for amyloid only the minimum exposure to these solutions required for resin removal should be used. Janes[9] reported successful resin removal and amyloid staining after 5 min exposure to saturated alcoholic sodium hydroxide.

### *1. Solutions*

Alcoholic sodium chloride-hydroxide
Stock solution
Saturated sodium chloride in 80% alcohol
Working solution

| | |
|---|---|
| Stock solution | 50 mℓ |
| 1% aqueous sodium hydroxide | 0.5 mℓ |

Mix and filter, use within 15 min

Congo red
Stock solution
Saturated congo red in 80% alcohol saturated with sodium chloride
Working solution

| | |
|---|---|
| Stock solution | 50 mℓ |
| 1% aqueous sodium hydroxide | 0.5 mℓ |

### *2. Technique*

1. Bring sections to water
2. Stain nuclei with Harris's or Carrazi's hematoxylin, differentiate, and blue
3. Treat with the alcoholic sodium chloride-hydroxide solution for 20 min drain
4. Stain with the congo red mixture for 20 min; rinse in alcohol
5. Dehydrate, clear, and mount.

### *3. Results*

| | |
|---|---|
| Eosinophils, amyloid, elastin | Dull red |
| Nuclei | Blue |
| Background | Clear |

When viewed in a polarizing microscope between crossed polaroids, amyloid stained with congo red exhibits an apple green birefringence.

## L. Bowie's Neutral Stain for Juxtaglomerular Cells[8]

Fixation in Helly's fluid is recommended.

### *1. Solutions*

2.5% aqueous potassium dichromate

Bowie's solution

Dissolve 1 g of Biebrich scarlet in 250 mℓ of distilled water and filter. Dissolve 2 g ethyl violet in 500 mℓ distilled water. Filter a small amount at a time of the latter solution into the Biebrich scarlet solution until a precipitate is formed. The end-point is reached when a small amount of the mixture placed on a No. 1 filter paper shows no coloration other than that of the precipitate. Filter the mixture and dry the precipitate in the filter paper. Finally dissolve 0.2 g of the dried precipitate in 20 mℓ of alcohol and use. There is normally enough precipitate to make 100 mℓ of stain.

### *2. Technique*

1. Bring the sections to water and remove any mercury precipitate
2. Mordant in the potassium dichromate solution overnight at 40°C
3. Wash well in tap water, then in distilled water
4. Stain with the Bowie's solution, diluted by adding 10 to 15 drops to 100 mℓ of 20% alcohol; leave overnight at room temperature
5. Drain and blot dry; remove excess stain by dipping in two changes of acetone
6. Differentiate in equal parts of xylene and clove oil until the section is an overall red or reddish-purple color, with any elastin picked out as blue-purple fibers
7. Rinse in xylene and mount in synthetic medium

### *3. Results*

| | |
|---|---|
| Juxtaglomerular granules, elastin | Blue-purple |
| Renal parenchyma | Red-magenta |

Although this method is rather time consuming we have found it preferable and more reliable than simpler procedures such as PAS-aldehyde fuchsin, thioflavine T fluorescence, and crystal violet methods.[8,10] A rapid crystal violet procedure is given as a screening stain for EM blocks.

We have found the above methods to be successful with both plastic and paraffin sections. Fixation has an important influence on staining properties and the Duboscq-Brasil fixative (Chapter 2) gives the best overall results. If other fixatives must be employed, staining may be enhanced by post-fixing the tissue in Duboscq-Brazil solution.

This can be done prior to embedding (Chapter 2) or the sections can be treated with the fixative for 1 hr before staining (or with saturated aqueous picric acid at 50°C for 30 min). An alternative method for enhancing the staining of epoxy-resin embedded sections was devised by Stoeckel.[11] This involves post-fixation with a dichromate-formalin mixture and subsequent oxidation with permanganate. Although originally devised to enhance aldehyde-fuchsin stains, Maxwell[12] has employed this technique with slight modifications to generally improve staining results with epoxy-resin embedded tissues. The details are given below for those who wish to try the method.

**Post-fixing mixture** —

| | |
|---|---|
| Potassium dichromate | 3 g |
| Formalin (37 to 40%) | 25 mℓ |
| Acetic acid | 5 mℓ |
| Distilled water | 70 mℓ |

Sections were left in this mixture for 1 hr at room temperature after the resin is removed and the section is rinsed in water.

**Oxidation solution** — 2.5% potassium permanganate in distilled water. After post-fixation sections were placed in this solution for 15 min at room temperature. The sections were finally bleached in 1% oxalic acid for 15 min at room temperature and then well washed in tap water. These procedures are not recommended prior to silver staining methods.

## VII. SPECIAL PROCEDURES

### A. Transfer of Material Originally Embedded in Paraffin into Plastic

This procedure is easily carried out and is occasionally useful to enable thinner sections of higher resolution to be obtained.

1. With a warm razor blade carefully cut from the wax block the tissue (or part of the tissue) that is to be transferred.
2. Place this in a large excess (10 × the tissue volume) of xylene and leave until the residual wax has dissolved.
3. Wash in two changes of fresh xylene — 10 min in each change.
4. Re-embed in Spurr's resin* by treating as follows:
   50% xylene/50% resin for 30 min,
   100% resin for 60 min.
   Embed in fresh resin and polymerize overnight at 70°C.

If it is preferred to re-embed in glycol methacrylate, after the final wash in xylene rinse in absolute alcohol and then proceed as follows:

| | |
|---|---|
| 50% GMA/alcohol | 15 min |
| 100% GMA | 15 min |
| Complete GMA mixture** | 30 min |
| Embed in capsules using fresh mixture and polymerize at 40°C | |

* EPON or ARALDITE may be used as alternative but less satisfactory resins.

** See Chapter 8 for details of the GMA mixture and the polymerization process.

**B. Optical Microscopy of Material Processed for Electron Microscopy**

It may sometimes be necessary to examine material processed for EM with the optical microscope. Insufficient glomeruli may be present in the biopsy portion processed for optical microscopy or the EM portion may contain material of particular interest. Sections of the EM block (0.25 to 1 $\mu$m) can be obtained in the usual manner (Chapter 4, Section II.A) and mounted on slides. Considerable information can then be gained from the standard Richardson's staining method (Chapter 4, Section II.A). However, if the usual optical staining techniques are preferred, special treatment is required. The epoxy embedment may be removed with sodium hydroxide or methoxide (Section IV). It is then necessary to remove osmium fixation residues before the tissue can be stained. This is conveniently done by treating the sections with 1% periodic acid for 30 min at room temperature. Following this step, the sections are washed in water and then stained by any of the methods given earlier. Note that no further oxidation is required for the PAS and silver methenamine methods.

The results obtained from sections treated in this way will not be as satisfactory as those from correctly embedded material; staining will be less intense and less selective.

## REFERENCES

1. **Churg, J. and Graham, E.**, Application of thin sections to problems of renal pathology, *J. Mt. Sinai Hosp. N.Y.*, 24, 736, 1957.
2. **Janes, R. B.**, A review of three resin processing techniques applicable to light microscopy, *Med. Lab. Sci.*, 36, 249, 1979.
3. **Agodoa, L., Striker, G., and Chi, E.**, Glycol methacrylate embedding of renal biopsy specimens for light microscopy, *Am. J. Clin. Pathol.*, 64, 655, 1975.
4. **Culling, C. F. A.**, *Handbook of Histological and Histochemical Techniques*, 3rd ed., Butterworths, London, 1974.
5. **Bennett, H. S., Wyrick, A. D., Lee, S. W., and McNeil, J. H., Jr.**, Science and art in preparing tissues embedded in plastic for light microscopy with special reference to glycol methacrylate, glass knives and simple stains, *Stain Technol.*, 51, 71, 1976.
6. **Spurr, A.**, A low-viscosity epoxy resin embedding medium for electron microscopy, *J. Ultrastruct. Res.*, 26, 31, 1969.
7. **Gamble, C. N.**, Periodic acid-Schiff-light green stain to detect glomerular protein deposits by routine light microscopy, *Am. J. Clin. Pathol.*, 63, 310, 1975.
8. **Cook, H. C.**, *Manual of Histological Demonstration Techniques*, Butterworths, London, 1974.
9. **Lendrum, A. C., Fraser, D. S., Slidders, W., and Henderson, R.**, Studies on the character and staining of fibrin, *J. Clin. Pathol.*, 15, 401, 1962.
10. **Harada, K.**, Rapid demonstration of juxtaglomerular granules with alcoholic crystal violet, *Stain Technol.*, 45, 71, 1970.
11. **Stoeckel, M. E., Porte, A., and Dellman, H. D.**, Selective staining of neurosecretory material in semithin epoxy sections by Gomori's aldehyde fuchsin, *Stain Technol.*, 47, 81, 1972.
12. **Maxwell, M. H.**, Two rapid and simple methods used for the removal of resins from 1.0$\mu$ thick epoxy sections, *J. Microsc. (Oxford)*, 112, 253, 1978.

Chapter 4

# ELECTRON MICROSCOPY

**David E. Allen and John P. Dowling**

## TABLE OF CONTENTS

## I. INTRODUCTION

The various preparative techniques for transmission electron microscopy (EM) have the aim of enabling ultrathin sections of tissue to be obtained. In order to achieve good resolution in the electron image the specimen thickness must be of the order of 800 Å or less. This necessitates that the tissue be embedded in a medium which will provide sufficient physical support for such thin sections to be cut. The embedment should also provide stability for the tissue in the rigorous conditions that exist in the electron microscope. In general, these provisions have been net by using plastic resins as embedding media. Tissue is infiltrated with a liquid embedding medium which is then polymerized to produce a solid block. Three main types of embedding media are in general use: epoxy resins, polyester resins, and methacrylates.

The epoxy resins are the most widely used since they are readily available, section well, and undergo little volume change on polymerization. Polyester resins also have excellent properties, but they are less readily available and some of the components are not stable during storage. Methacrylates are useful for immuno-EM, cytochemistry, and light microscopy (Chapter 2), but they are not well suited for general EM. Their polymerization may be uneven and the polymers are less stable under electron bombardment. Because of the wide usage of epoxy resins, we will confine our discussion to examples of these materials found useful in processing renal biopsies. An account and details of use of polyester resins and methacrylates may be found in Glauert.[1]

Before fixed tissue can be infiltrated with epoxy resin it is necessary to replace the water present in the tissue with a solvent miscible with the resin monomers. This dehydration is usually carried out by transferring the tissue through increasing concentrations of ethanol or acetone. Acetone is the preferred solvent as it is more miscible with the resin monomers, although following the use of uranyl acetate as a third fixative, it is advisable to begin dehydration with alcohol/water mixtures to present the precipitation of uranium salts. If only ethanol is available, exchange of this solvent with propylene oxide prior to infiltration is desirable. This epoxide solvent is fully miscible with epoxy resins and small amounts of residual solvent are incorporated into the polymeric resin. Propylene oxide should be handled with care as it is highly volatile, inflammable, and toxic.

It is important that the solvents used in the final stages of dehydration and during infiltration be free of water. Even small amounts of water will lead to poor infiltration, difficult sectioning, and poor ultrastructural preservation. Absolute ethanol (not commercial spirit) and a good grade of propylene oxide usually satisfy these requirements, but bottles should be used as soon as possible after opening and kept tightly stoppered. Acetone absorbs water very readily and even good commercial grades may contain appreciable quantities of water. This is most easily removed by adding anhydrous copper sulfate to the solvent. A 1-cm layer of this salt added to a 500-mℓ bottle of acetone will remove any water present and also any absorbed while the bottle is in use. The action of this dehydrating agent is rather slow and it should be added to the solvent some 24 hr before the bottle is used. It is preferable to purchase the dehydrating solvent in bottles of 500 mℓ rather than a larger size so that a bottle is used fairly quickly once opened.

## II. EMBEDDING

We shall confine our description of embedding procedures for EM to methods using the epoxy resins EPON 812 and ARALDITE CY212. (EPON and ARALDITE are trade names for epoxy resins originally developed by the Shell Chemical Conpany and Ciba Products Corp., respectively. These terms are now in common usage.) However, it should be noted that the Spurr's low-viscosity resin used for light microscopy may also be used for electron microscopy. DURCUPAN ACM* is a product of Fluka (Switzerland) which is similar to ARALDITE CY212 (Ciba) and DURCUPAN may be used in place of ARALDITE in the methods given below. EPON is available from a number of suppliers (see Appendix).

Both of these epoxy-resins produce polymers that section well and the sections have good stability in the electron beam. The ARALDITE polymer is somewhat easier to section and it is the most stable due to a higher degree of cross-linking. However, this cross-linking does reduce stain penetration and longer staining times are required for tissues embedded in ARALDITE. The silver methenamine method (Section XI) does not work at all on ARALDITE sections and if this technique is to be used, EPON embedding should be employed. Mollenhauer[2] recommended mixtures of EPON and ARALDITE for embedding and suggested that the mixture combined the favorable properties of both resins. However, the silver methenamine stain will not penetrate this mixed polymer either and we have found ARALDITE preferable for routine work.

Epoxy-resin components are supplied in cans or bottles which may be stored indefinitely at room temperature as long as they are kept tightly sealed. Up to four components may be supplied: the epoxy component (resin), the hardener (acid anhydride), the accelerator (organic amine), and the plasticizer (dibutyl phthalate). Particular care is needed to protect the hardener from moisture. All epoxy-resin components should be handled with care as they are toxic and may cause dermatitis in susceptible persons.

* Fluka also produces a water-soluble form of DURCUPAN (usually termed DURCUPAN — water soluble); this is not recommended for routine EM.

When mixing the monomer components to form the embedding medium, accurate measuring of the monomers is important as even small variations in the ratio of resin to hardener and accelerator will affect the sectioning properties of the polymer. Because of the high viscosity of the monomers, it is difficult to measure out the components by volume. An easier and more accurate procedure is to measure the monomers by weighing. Only dry apparatus should be used for mixing the resin components and it is advantageous to briefly warm the apparatus before use to drive off any moisture present. In the case of glassware, this is conveniently done by running flasks, etc. through a bunsen flame.

Glassware contaminated with epoxy-resins may be cleaned by rinsing with technical grade acetone to remove most of the resin. After a thorough wash in water, residual resin is removed by soaking in chromic acid (see Chapter 3). It is important to ensure that *all* organic solvents are washed away before the glassware is placed in the acid. Because of the dangerous nature of chromic acid, some laboratories prefer to use only acetone and hot, soapy water for cleaning or, alternatively, disposable apparatus is used. Resin must be washed off apparatus as soon as possible and certainly before polymerization occurs as it is then almost impossible to remove.

Waste resin from infiltration steps should not be poured into sinks or drains as there is considerable danger of blocking pipes. It is better to collect the material in a can or jar and allow it to polymerize over a period of weeks . This results in an inert solid which is more easily disposed of.

To prepare the monomer mixture, appropriate quantities of resin hardener and plasticizer (see below) are carefully weighed into a dry flask. These components are mixed to form a homogenous solution. With small quantities of monomers (up to 40 g), this mixing can be achieved by shaking, but larger quantities will require mechanical or magnetic stirring. Mixing is facilitated by gentle warming of the components to reduce their viscosity. However, the temperature of the mix should not exceed 40 to 50°C. When thoroughly mixed, these components are allowed to cool and the correct quantity of accelerator is added. This is rapidly mixed into the resin-hardener mixture. As the accelerator components of both EPON and ARALDITE are of lower viscosity they may be measured with a graduated disposable syringe (1 mℓ). As the monomer mixture slowly polymerizes at room temperature, only sufficient mixture for immediate needs should be prepared. It is convenient to prepare one batch of mixture for infiltration and then a fresh batch for final embedding. It is possible to store the mixed monomers for periods of 24 to 48 hr in a refrigerator. Containers must be tightly sealed to prevent the entry of water and the mixture must be allowed to reach room temperature before opening to prevent condensation from affecting the resin.

## III. RESIN MIXTURES

### A. ARALDITE

| | |
|---|---|
| Resin component | 5 g |
| Hardener | 5 g |
| Plasticizer (dibutyl phthalate) | 1 mℓ |
| Mix as described above and add accelerator | 0.2 mℓ |

### B. DURCUPAN

1. Component A
2. Component B
3. Mix as described above and add Component C

This mixture usually gives a polymer that is satisfactory for EM without addition of component D (plasticizer — dibutyl phthalate). If a softer resin is required, small amounts of D may be added (e.g., 0.5 to 1.0 mℓ). An increase in the ratio of B to A will produce a harder resin.

### C. EPON

| | |
|---|---|
| EPON 812 | 16 g |
| Dodecyl succinic anhydride | 8 g |
| Nadic methyl anhydride | 9.2 g |
| Mix as described above and add DMP-30 accelerator | 0.48 mℓ |

The hardness of EPON polymers can be varied over a wide range by changing the ratio of the monomers to one another. For full details consult Polysciences data sheet No. 116 (supplied with all Polysciences EPON kits). The above mixture is satisfactory for renal biopsies.

Tissue specimens ane infiltrated with resin by soaking in increasing concentrations of the mixed monomers dissolved in acetone or propylene oxide. If the infiltration and embedding process cannot be completed in 1 day, we have found it advantageous to leave the tissue, in the resin mixture, in a vacuum desiccator overnight. Tissue treated in this manner routinely sections more readily.[3] Possibly the vacuum aids infiltration and the desiccant prevents absorption of moisture by the resin. Only a mild desiccant such as anhydrous sodium sulfate is needed as the drying agent. Suitable infiltration procedures are given below.

It is preferable to rotate the specimen containers during infiltration as this greatly aids penetration of the resin mixture. A simple rotating stage can be constructed by drilling holes of a size which will hold the specimen containers in a wooden disk. The disk is then clamped to the spindle of a low-speed motor which is attached to a bench or positioned on a stand. Alternatively, rotating stages are available commercially. We routinely use disposable glass vials of 2 to 5 mℓ capacity for processing specimens. Vials made of plastic (polypropylene, not polystyrene) are also suitable if propylene oxide is not used as an intermediate solvent. The same vial can be used throughout the processing schedule up to the final embedding step. A variety of molds for final embedding are available ranging from gelatin capsules to specially shaped capsules and trays which reduce the amount of trimming required prior to microtomy (see Appendix). We have found small aluminum weighing dishes of approximately 1½ in. in diameter to be a cheap and convenient source of molds. These dishes are thin enough for the metal to be marked by a pencil and the dish can be marked into separate areas for different biopsies, each of which can be numbered. The marks of the dish appear on the resin block after polymerization. Individual biopsies may be sawed from the solid block and filed in small boxes. Another low-cost alternative is to use plastic vial caps as molds for individual specimens. A paper label can be incorporated in the mold (using pencil or indelible ink markings) to aid identification.

Final polymerization of the epoxy-resin is achieved by placing the molds in an oven at 70 to 80°C for at least 12 hr. Small ovens are commercially available for this purpose, but any oven that can reliably maintain this temperature is suitable. It is advantageous to leave the molds in the oven for longer than 12 hr. The cutting properties of the blocks improve significantly over 2 to 3 days. Tissue embedded in resin is stable indefinitely at room temperature and blocks may be stored in any convenient filing system.

## IV. DEHYDRATION INFILTRATION AND EMBEDDING

### A. Normal Schedule

The times for each step will vary according to the size of the tissue specimens being processed. Thin or very small specimens can be processed rather quickly while larger pieces will require longer periods.

1. Dehydrate in 30, 50, and 70% alcohol or acetone for 15 to 30 min in each. Tissues may be stored overnight in the refrigerator in 70% alcohol or acetone. Alcohol is preferred for initial dehydration when the tissue has been treated with uranyl acetate.
2. Dehydrate in 90% acetone and three changes of dry acetone for 30 min each.
3. Infiltrate with resin by passing through increasing concentrations of resin in dry acetone:

| Parts resin | plus | Parts dry acetone | Time (min) |
|---|---|---|---|
| 1 | | 4 | 20—30 |
| 2 | | 3 | 20—30 |
| 3 | | 2 | 20—30 |
| 4 | | 1 | 20—30 |

4. Undiluted resin 1 to 2 hr; tissues can be stored in a vacuum desiccator overnight at this stage.
5. Undiluted resin for 2 to 3 hr at 35°C.
6. Embed tissues in gelatine capsules or molds, place in a 45°C oven for a few hours then transfer to a 70 to 80°C oven and leave for at least 12 hr to harden.

### B. Compressed Schedule

1. Dehydrate for 3 min each in 30, 50, and 70% alcohol
2. 90% acetone 5 min
3. Absolute acetone 3 × 5 min
4. 1 part resin plus 2 parts acetone for 10 min
5. 2 parts resin plus 1 part acetone for 10 min
6. Undiluted resin for 20 min
7. Embed and cure in 90°C oven for at least 1 hr or overnight. The longer the curing time, the better the sectioning properties of the polymerized block.

Only small pieces of tissue should be processed using this schedule and the longer method is preferred when sufficient time is available.

A method for rapidly dehydrating tissue using dimethoxypropane was described by Muller and Jacks.[4] In this method, the tissue is simply immersed in acidified dimethoxypropane for minutes. Water in the tissue reacts with the propane derivative to form acetone and methanol and in the process the tissue is dehydrated. We have tested this method, but in our hands it was difficult to obtain uniform dehydration of renal biopsies and the subsequent infiltration of resin was poor. We cannot therefore recommend the method.

It is important that all infiltration and embedding steps be carried out carefully. Poor processing will lead to specimens which cannot be sectioned or the sections will disin-

**Table 1**
**COMMON EMBEDDING FAULTS AND THEIR POSSIBLE CAUSE**

| | |
|---|---|
| Blocks too soft | Wrong component mix, polymerization temperature too low |
| Blocks too brittle | Wrong component mix; add less hardener or include dibutyl phthalate as a plasticizer |
| Blocks discoloured | Old accelerator — change to fresh bottle |
| Blocks section poorly and thick (1 μm) sections react weakly with Richardsons stain | Polymer formed with hydrated hardener; see above method |

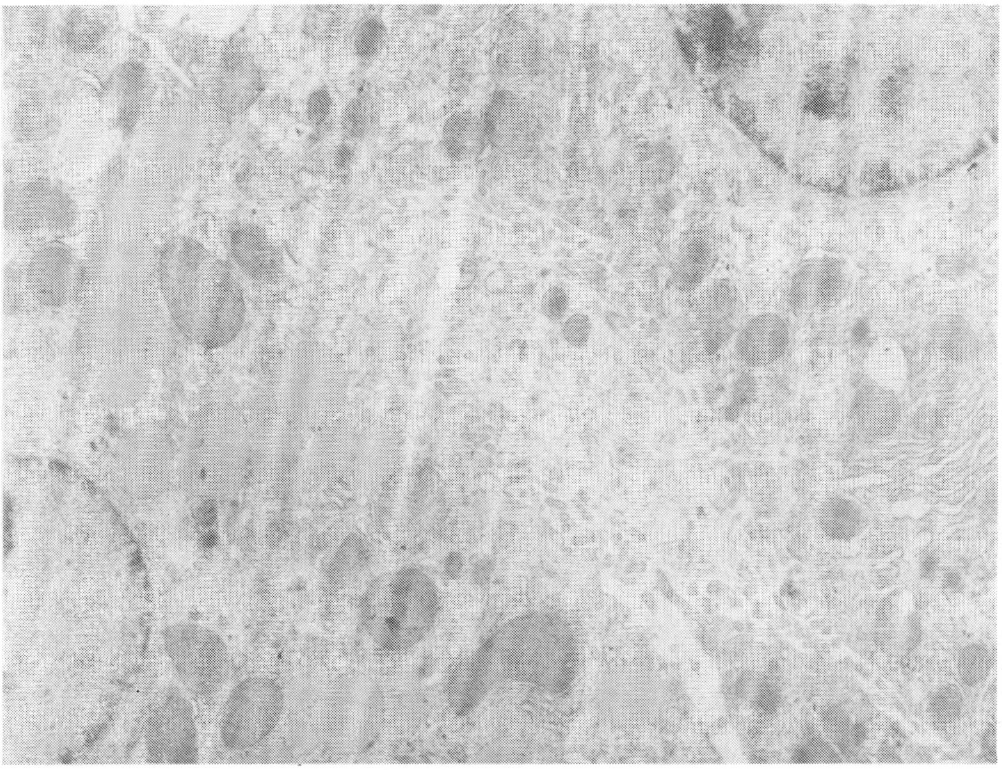

FIGURE 1. Rat liver tissue. Fixation: PIPES buffered glutaraldehyde and paraformaldehyde, post-fixed in Dalton's fixative. Staining: uranyl acetate in the block and uranyl acetate and lead citrate on the grid. (Magnification × 15,000 shown at 65%.) Poorly infiltrated tissue producing a soft block which has resulted in chatter during sectioning.

tegrate on handling (see Table 1). Material which is not properly embedded will not yield satisfatory micrographs (Figure 1). This can be disastrous when biopsy material is irreplaceable or when an urgent report is required. A common embedding problem arises from the use of hydrated hardeners. Improperly stored hardeners will readily absorb moisture and this interferes with the polymerization process. This problem is to be suspected when thin sections of tissue disintegrate into small fragments upon contact with the water in knife trough.

### C. Rescue Method for Poorly Embedded Tissues

McNelly and Hinds[5] have published a method for rescuing tissue suffering from this fault. The technique is also suitable for reclaiming material which was insufficiently dehydrated (usually through the use of "wet" dehydrating agents). Ten-micron sections of the poorly embedded tissue are cut and placed in an aluminum weighing dish. The sections are covered with distilled water and the dish heated on a hot plate until the water has evaporated, leaving the sections adhering to the bottom. Fresh embedding media is then added to the dishes and they are placed in a vacuum desiccator overnight and subsequently transferred to a 60°C oven for 48 hr. Following this procedure the tissue can frequently be thin-sectioned without difficulty and the ultrastructure is much improved.

## V. ULTRAMICROTOMY

It is not within the scope of this book to give a detailed account of ultramicrotome operation. Sectioning procedures vary according to the machine being used and the best source of data on any particular instrument is usually the manufacturer's instruction book. Similarly, basic details of ultrathin sectioning technique are provided by most microtome manufacturers and an excellent review is given by Reid.[6] We shall, however, give details of some methods which we have found to aid sectioning and discuss some of the problems occurring in the ultramicrotomy of biopsy material.

In general, properly embedded renal tissue poses few problems in ultramicrotomy and sections showing silver-gold interference colors are readily obtained. Glass knives are adequate for biopsy work, although in the hands of a skilled operator better sections will be produced by a diamond knife. If diamond knives are to be used, it is best for an individual operator to be given responsibility for a particular knife. Diamond knives are delicate and must be cleaned regularly according to the manufacturer's instructions. If neglected, a diamond knife will produce sections which are greatly inferior to those obtainable from glass knives.

Usually the glomerular areas of renal cortex are of most interest in the EM of biopsy specimens. In order to find these areas the biopsy samples must be sectioned, and the sections examined at regular intervals by optical microscopy until a glomerulus is located. The specimen block is then trimmed so that the glomerulus is favorably oriented for ultrathin sectioning. This preliminary sectioning may be done on the ultramicrotome, although some manufacturers (e.g., LKB) produce special instruments for this purpose. The sections are generally cut at 0.5 to 2.0 $\mu$m and a representative section is mounted on a glass slide for examination after every 20 to 30 $\mu$m. It is advisable not to attempt to section epoxy blocks at thicknesses in excess of 2 $\mu$m as tearing of the tissue may result in the formation of holes in the surface of the block. These "thick" sections are easily mounted on slides by picking up the section from the knife trough with a clean wire loop and transferring it to a drop of water on the slide. The section will readily free itself from the loop and remain floating in the water droplet. If this does not happen, the loop surface is probably contaminated and should be cleaned by heating to redness in a flame. The section is dried down onto the slide by careful heating over a small flame or on a hot plate. Resin sections can be examined unstained by phase-contrast microscopy or they may be simply stained with toluidine blue or methylene blue. These dyes act most strongly in alkaline solution and a useful mixture with excellent staining properties is that of Richardson.[7] The stain consists of equal volumes of 1% aqueous azure II and 1% methylene blue dissolved in 1% aqueous borax. Staining is carried out by adding a drop of stain over the section on the slide and warming gently (flame or hot-plate) for 30 sec to 1 min, although tissues treated with uranyl acetate may require a longer staining time. After rinsing with water, the slide is blotted dry and examined with a microscope. For viewing purposes, a coverslip is not required, but if the sections are to be kept, a coverslip may be mounted oven the dry section with either liquid resin mixture or a synthetic mounting medium. Richardson's stain acts as a general stain and most tissue components are colored to some extent, enabling ready identification of areas of interest. In fact, sections stained in this manner show a resemblance to low-power electron micrographs. It has been suggested that this staining method may even reduce the need for EM. Glomerular protein deposits are often readily visible and many more glomeruli can be examined than is possible by EM.

**A. Summary of Richardson's Staining Procedure for Light Microscopy of EM Tissue**

*1. Stock Solutions*

(A) 1% Methylene blue in 1% aqueous borax solution.
(B) 1% Azure II in distilled water.

Mix equal quantities of A and B to prepare the working solution.

*2. Method*

1. Cut sections at 0.25 to 2μm with a glass knife. Transfer to a glass slide using wire loops.
2. Warm the slide on a hot plate or over a small flame until the section dries down on the slide.
3. Cover the section with a few drops of stain and warm gently for about 2 min (hot plate or flame).
4. Rinse off the stain and blot dry.
5. If necessary, apply a coverslip with liquid resin or synthetic mounting media.

If extra color differentiation of tissue structures is preferred, the basic-fuchsin-crystal violet sequence described by Lee and Hopper may be used.[8] This technique is given as a rapid stain for localizing the juxtaglomerular apparatus prior to EM sectioning. The authors claim that the method is superior to monochromatic methods for this purpose and gives excellent contrast and intensity.

**B. Rapid Stain for Juxtaglomerular Granules or a Polychromic Method for General Morphology**

*1. Solutions*

| | | |
|---|---|---|
| A. | 30% alcohol | 100 mℓ |
| | Basic fuchsin | 1 g |
| | Aniline | 1 mℓ |
| | Phenol | 1 g |
| B. | Absolute alcohol | 10 mℓ |
| | Crystal violet | 5 g |
| | Aniline | 2 mℓ |
| | Distilled water | 88 mℓ |

Dissolve the dye in the alcohol and then add the other components. Filter the solution.

*2. Technique*

1. Cut sections (approximately 0.5μm) and dry onto the slide as in Steps 1 and 2, above, EPON sections may require albumin-coated slides to ensure adherence.
2. Agitate slides in xylene for 15 sec then for 15 sec each in 95% and 80% alcohol then in water.

3. Immerse in Solution A for 20 to 30 sec.
4. Rinse gently in water to remove excess stain.
5. Immerse in Solution B for 20 to 30 sec.
6. Rinse in water to remove excess stain and dry on hot plate or over small flame.
7. Apply coverslip if required with liquid resin or synthetic medium.

*3. Results*

| | |
|---|---|
| Granules of juxtaglomerular apparatus | Intense dark blue |
| Elastic and connective tissues | Pale blue |
| Basement membranes, red blood cells, mitochondria and brush border of tubules | Dark red |
| Other cytoplasmic features | Pale red |

Once a glomerulus has been located, the specimen block is further trimmed so that the block face has a minimum of surplus tissue and especially a minimum of empty plastic. This is not always easy as glomeruli frequently occur at the edges of the tissue and some empty plastic may have to be included in the final block face. This may create sectioning difficulties because of the differences in hardness of tissue and plastic. In some cases the problem is eased by reorienting the block in the specimen holder so that the empty plastic appears in a different position during sectioning. Reorientation also helps when chatter occurs and when alternatively thick and thin sections are cut.

When the block is ready for thin-sectioning, if it is not absolutely essential to collect all the sections from a tissue block it is a good idea to discard the first few ultrathin sections as they will have imperfections from the trimming process and also holes left in the block from the thick-sectioning process.

One of the more difficult tasks in ultramicrotomy is that of transferring the cut sections from the knife trough onto a metal specimen grid. The best of sections are useless if they cannot be successfully collected on a grid. For most purposes copper specimen grids are used, but some cytochemical procedures (e.g., the silver methenamine stain) demand the use of other materials due to the chemical activity of copper. In these cases grids of gold, nickel, or stainless steel may be used. We have found the latter to be preferable. Gold is expensive and nickel grids can be difficult to handle in the vicinity of microscopes as they attach themselves firmly to forceps, etc. which have become magnetized by the lens fields. Whatever the nature of the grids it is important that they be clean. Grids coated with a film of grease are very hydrophobic and sections will tend to move away from them. This results in the sections being "chased around the knife trough" when attempts are made to collect them. This frequently leads to destruction of the sections. Grids are easily degreased by rinsing in acetone; this procedure also appears to remove surface oxide layers and sections attach most readily to freshly cleaned grids. For this reason, it is desirable to clean the working collection of grids at frequent intervals. For routine biopsy work with properly embedded tissue it is not necessary to use grids coated with a carbon or plastic film. Sections of material embedded in EPON or ARALDITE and showing silver-gold interference colors should have sufficient stability to be used on uncoated 200-mesh grids. However, if grids of larger mesh size are used or if the wide-field technique of Yang and Morrison is attempted (see below), coating may be required. Methods of preparing plastic and carbon films are given below.

Even clean uncoated grids tend to be hydrophilic in nature causing sections to be repelled from them during collection from the knife trough. This results in sections attaching irregularly to the grid with consequent risk of folding. This problem can be overcome by immersing individual grids, immediately before use, in a very dilute solution of bovine serum albumin (BSA). This protein acts as a wetting agent and treated grids will not repel sections. This enables sections to be positioned as required on the grid surface. A solution of 2 mg of albumin in 5 mℓ of distilled water is adequate for this purpose. The very small amount of albumin transferred to the knife trough as each section is picked up has no ill effects. However, it is important that the albumin solution be freshly prepared each day to prevent growth of microorganisms. Residual albumin on the specimen grids can cause sections to detach from the specimen grids during staining operations. This is easily overcome by exposing the grids to glutaraldehyde *vapor* for 5 to 10 min. This destroys the wetting properties of the albumin, but has no visible effect upon the sections. The operation is conveniently carried out by placing the grids in a closed vessel containing a little 25% glutaraldehyde solution.

## C. Methods for the Preparation of Support Films

### *1. Plastic Films*

The specimen grids to be coated are placed on a piece of copper gauze (30 mesh, 32 gauge) that is bent at right angles at the edges. The gauze and grids are then placed in a dish filled with a stopcock which is filled with distilled water.

One drop of a 0.5 to 1% solution of formvar in ethylene dichloride (or 2% nitrocellulose in amyl acetate) is placed on the end of a clean microscope slide and spread over the surface of the slide with a glass rod or the edge of another slide. The solvent will evaporate rapidly leaving a plastic film on the glass. Alternatively, a slide can be dipped in the formvar solution, drained, and allowed to dry at an angle. A raxor blade edge is run around the edges of the film and the slide is lowered into the dish of water containing the grids. The film should detach from the slide and remain floating on the water surface. If the film will not separate from the slide, the glass may be too clean. A further slide should be prepared after washing the glass with detergent and wiping dry without a rinse in water.

By running water out of the dish, the film will settle onto the grids. After drying, individual grids can be detached from the gauze.

### *2. Carbon Films*

Grids are first coated with a plastic film as described above and then placed in an evaporating unit. A 50 to 100 Å thick layer of carbon is evaporated onto the plastic coated grids. The traditional method of determining the thickness of the carbon layer is by observing a white porcelain tile placed in the evaporator and spotted with a drop of oil. The area of the tile not covered with oil will darken as carbon is evaporated onto it. A just detectable brown color represents a carbon thickness of approximately 50 Å while a chocolate brown deposit gives a thickness of about 100 Å.

Following carbon evaporation the plastic substrate is removed by placing the grids in a petri dish containing ethylene dichloride or amyl acetate. Carbon coatings can be made thinner than plastic films and are preferred when maximum quality or resolution is required.

Young and Morrison[9] have discussed a technique that provides a bridge between light and EM. Termed "wide-field microscopy", this method utilizes ultrathin sections mounted on slot-type grids coated with formvar support films. The intervention of the grid bars of conventional mesh grids is avoided and a continuous micrograph of large areas of the specimen (e.g., a whole glomerulus) can be obtained at scanning magnifications. The method provides micrographs which can be easily correlated with light microscope studies, but does demand a high degree of technical expertise and it is somewhat time consuming. Full technical details are provided in the authors' publication.

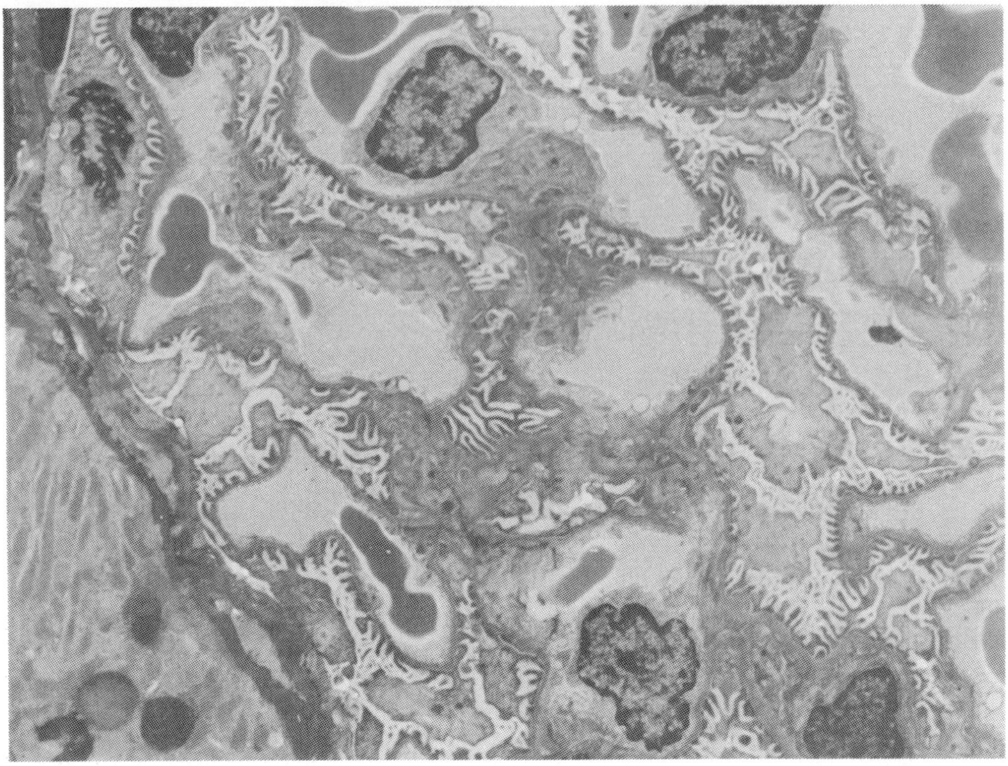

FIGURE 2. Rat kidney tissue. Fixation: PIPES buffered glutaraldehyde and paraformaldehyde. Staining: uranyl acetate in the block and uranyl acetate and lead citrate on the grid. (Magnification × 9300 shown at 65%.) Aldehyde fixation alone results in some loss of ultrastructural detail (compare Figures 4 and 7). Membranes particularly are less distinct but staining intensity is increased due to the absence of competition by osmium for stain-binding sites.

## VI. STAINING

A large number of staining techniques have now been developed for EM (for a review see References 10 and 11), although the EM examination of renal biopsy material will generally require the use of only a few of these. It is important to realize that the appearance of the electron microscope image depends greatly on the staining procedure used. In turn, the effects of staining reactions are dependent upon the earlier processing of the tissue. One has only to compare the appearance of tissue fixed only with glutaraldehyde to that of similar tissue fixed with a conventional double fixation sequence to appreciate this point (Figure 2). It is therefore desirable that a standardized processing and staining regime be used so that the comparison of biopsies is facilitated.

If a triple fixation sequence including osmium tetroxide and uranyl acetate fixation was employed, ultrathin sections of tissue will already show some contrast in the electron microscope (Figure 3). Such sections can be viewed and photographed without further staining. This process will be facilitated by using a small objective aperture (20μm and a low accelerating voltage (e.g., 60 kV). However, much improved results and easier appreciation of pathological changes will be possible if additional section staining procedures are used. The intensity of staining can be varied to suit individual preferences, but again it is emphasized that it is a good idea to standardize on the chosen procedure.

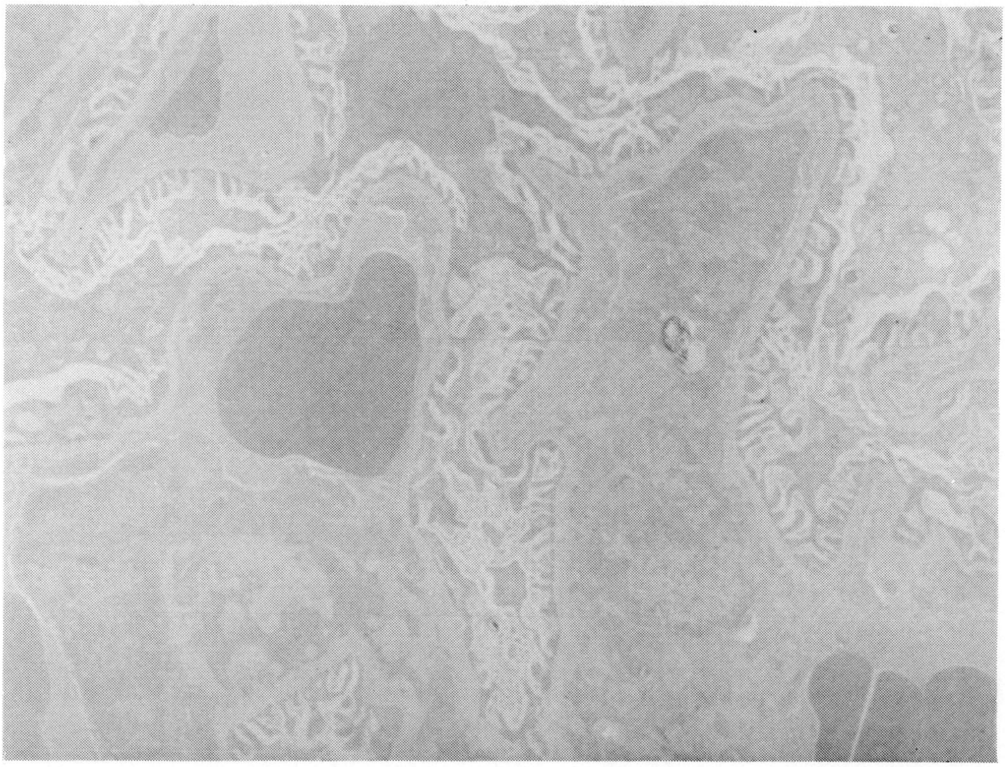

FIGURE 3. Rat kidney tissue. Fixation: PIPES buffered glutaraldehyde and paraformaldehyde, post-fixation with Dalton's fixative. Staining: uranyl acetate in the block only. (Magnification × 15,000 shown at 65%.) There is insufficient contrast for detailed study and the need to use a low accelerating voltage (40 kV) reduces resolution. Photographic enhancement of contrast results in increased prominence of knifemarks and other section faults.

Ultrathin sections mounted on specimen grids are readily stained by floating or immersing the grids in the staining solution. Floating has the advantage that any precipitate produced in the stain will tend to settle on the bottom of the container rather than on the sections. When the stain is in aqueous solution a particularly convenient technique is to place drops of stain on a sheet of dental wax contained in a shallow dish with a tight fitting lid. (When using lead stains the dish can also contain sodium hydroxide pellets to absorb atmospheric carbon dioxide.) The grids are easily floated (section side down) on the drops and several biopsies, each confined to individual drops, can be stained in this manner. The lower surface tension of nonaqueous solvents precludes the use of this method. When such solvents are used, the grids are immersed in stain contained in small glass or plastic petri dishes. Again, these are then placed in a closed vessel to prevent contamination.

After staining for the required time, the grids are rinsed in several changes of the stain solvent and placed on a filter paper to dry. The washing solvent can also be placed in small glass or plastic petri dishes. A particularly convenient type of dish is the six-well tissue culture dish manufactured by a number of suppliers (e.g., Disposable Products — see Appendix). Although intended to be disposable, these trays are easily rinsed for reuse. When rinsing the grids it is important that they not be held all the time with forceps. Invariably, a drop of stain is trapped between the forcep arms and unless the grid is released in the washing solution, this drop will remain in the forceps until the

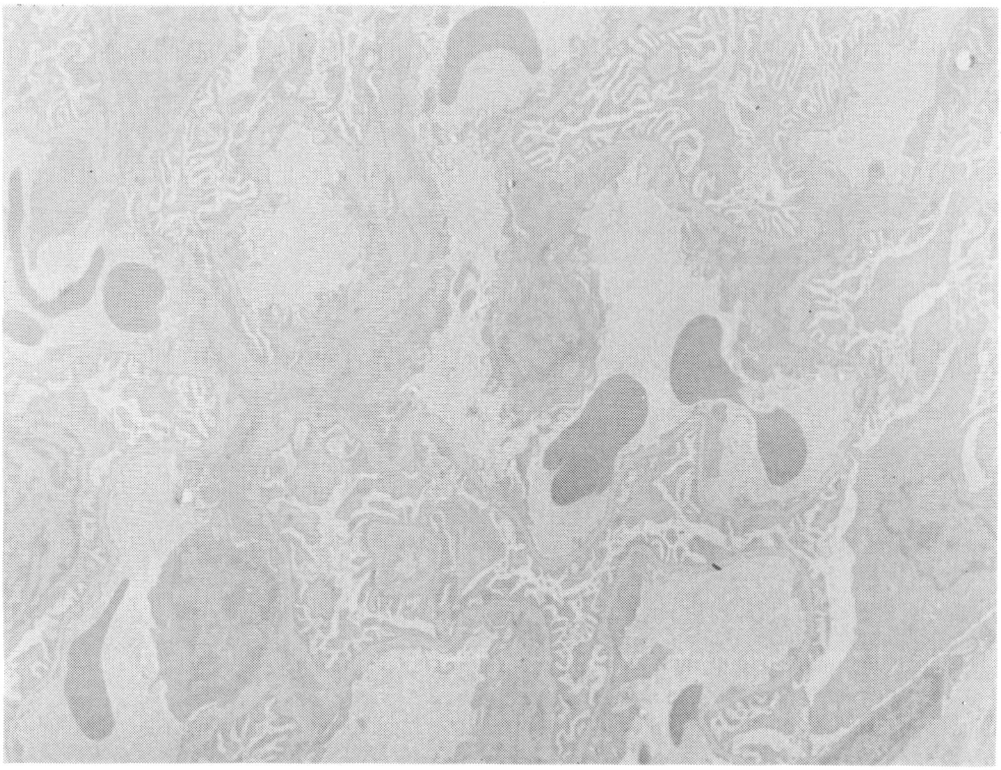

FIGURE 4. Rat kidney tissue. Fixation: PIPES buffered glutaraldehyde and paraformaldehyde, post-fixed in Dalton's fixative. Staining: uranyl acetate in the block and on the grid. (Magnification × 7800 shown at 65%.) Although grid staining with uranium increases contrast over that of Figure 3, the result is still inferior to combined grid staining with lead and uranium (Figures 7 and 8).

grid is placed on filter paper to dry. At this point any trapped stain will be released onto the grid causing contamination.

Treating the sections with solutions of uranium salts is a convenient way of producing additional contrast (Figure 4). Uranyl acetate, nitrate, and magnesium uranyl acetate have been used, but all produce similar results with renal biopsies. We routinely use uranyl acetate. Uranyl salts stain both nucleic acids and also proteins, binding probably occurring through the phosphate groups of the former and with the free amino groups of proteins. Solutions of uranyl acetate are readily prepared and are not subject to contamination by reaction with atmospheric carbon dioxide. The solutions are however photosensitive and should be used and kept in subdued light or in the dark. Also, they may form precipitates after standing for several weeks and any solutions showing a change in color or deposits should be discarded. It should be noted that uranium salts are toxic and radioactive. Care should be taken not to spill the material and wastes should be disposed of with care.

Staining with uranium may be carried out with solution of uranyl acetate in water, ethanol, or methanol. Methanolic solutions can be more concentrated and they produce more intense staining. However, the methanol can damage ultrathin sections, producing tearing and folding. Care must also be taken to avoid evaporation of the solvent or deposits will be produced on the sections (Figure 5). A compromise method is to use a saturated solution of uranyl acetate in 70% ethanol. This solution has a surface tension just sufficient to float grids and section damage usually does not occur. Staining intensity is greater than that achieved with aqueous solutions and this method is currently popular.

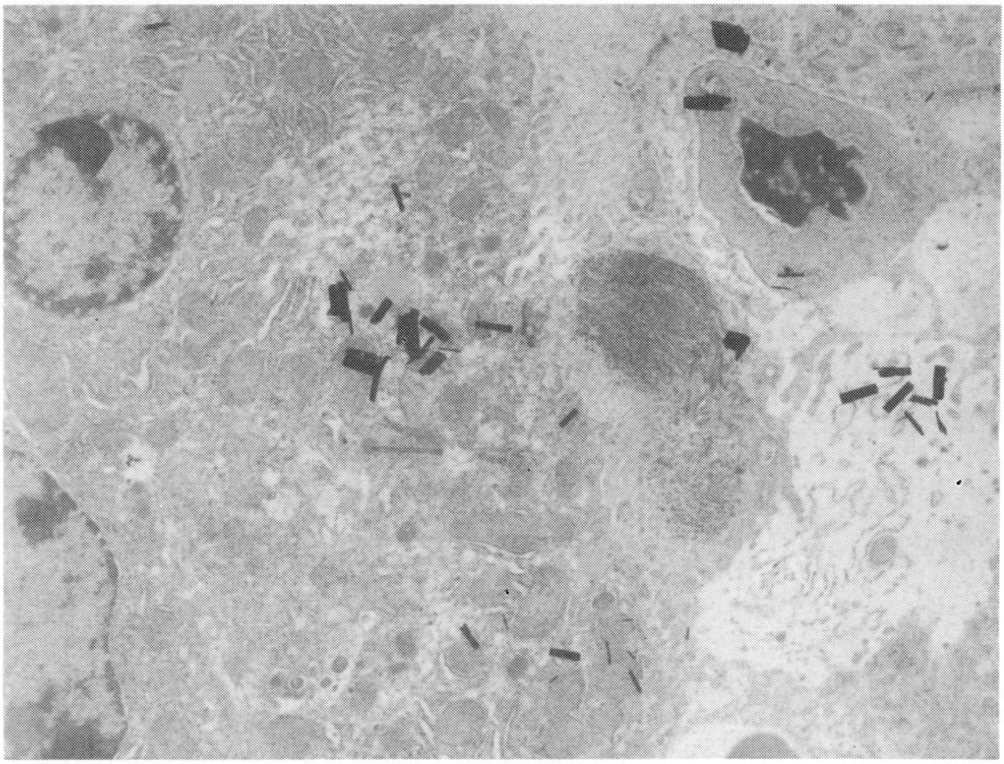

FIGURE 5. Rat liver tissue. Fixation: PIPES buffered glutaraldehyde and paraformaldehyde, post-fixed in Dalton's fixative. Staining: uranyl acetate in the block and uranyl acetate and lead citrate on the grid. (Magnification × 14,000 shown at 65%.) Poorly fixed and stained tissue; osmium deposits are again present (as Figure 6), and crystalline deposits of uranyl acetate obscure ultrastructural details.

Aqueous solutions of uranyl acetate overcome the disadvantages of organic solvents though the resulting staining is less intense. A 5% solution of the salt in water is suitable.

An alternative method of increasing overall contrast is to treat the sections with solutions of lead salts. The precise mechanism of lead staining is uncertain, but possibly involves two types of reactions with tissue.[12] In one of these lead is bound at site which gives a positive PAS reaction at the optical microscope level. This may be due to binding of lead to hydroxyl groups. In the other, lead is ionically bound to negatively charged osmium residues within the tissue. The result of these reactions is that lead solutions produce high contrast and stain many tissue components. Unfortunately, solutions of lead salts are particularly prone to contamination. The lead in solution reacts with atmospheric carbon dioxide to produce insoluble lead carbonate. This material precipitates on sections as a highly electron-dense "dirt" (Figure 6). In order to reduce the magnitude of this problem several workers have developed staining solutions in which lead ions are chelated by organic carboxylic acids. This reduces the rate of reaction with carbon dioxide. Fortunately, chemical groups naturally present in the tissue are able to compete for the chelated lead and so staining still occurs. The high pH of these mixtures aids staining as complexes containing several lead ions are formed. The most frequently used of these chelate stains is Reynolds "lead citrate".[13] This stain is readily prepared from stable ingredients and, provided that reasonable care is taken to prevent absorption of carbon dioxide, no contamination should occur. The solution should be kept in a closed vessel, preferably with a layer of hexane covering the surface of the stain, and staining

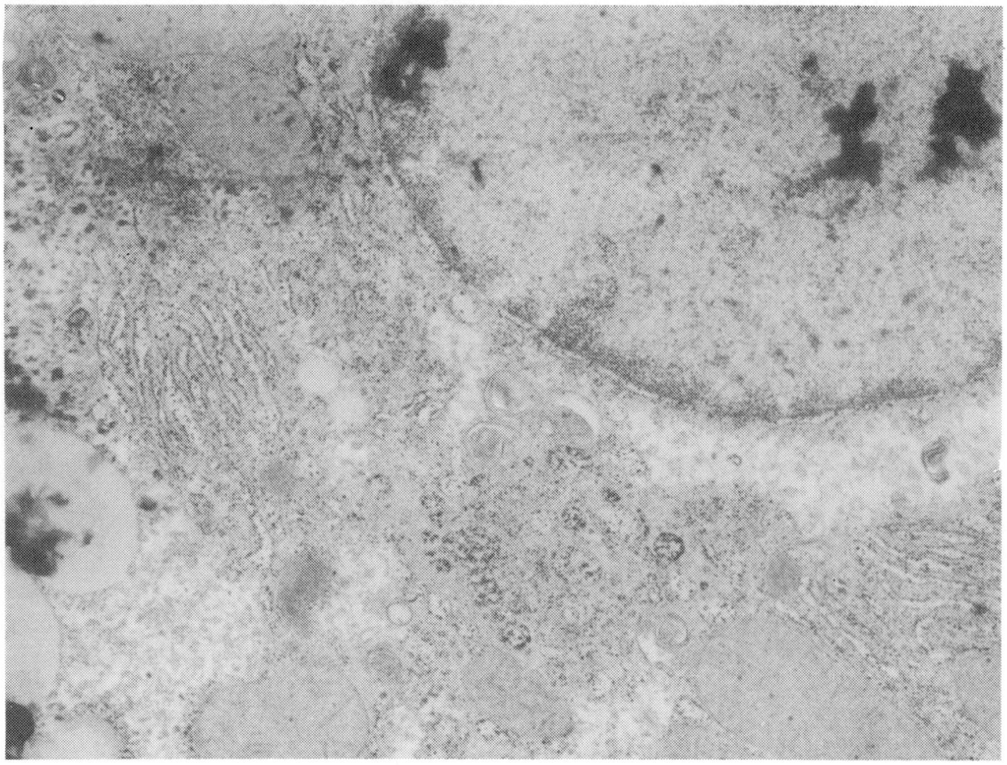

FIGURE 6. Rat liver tissue. Fixation: PIPES buffered glutaraldehyde and paraformaldehyde, post-fixed in Dalton's fixative. Staining: uranyl acetate in the block and uranyl acetate and lead citrate on the grid. (Magnification × 25,000 shown at 65%.) Poorly fixed and stained tissue; the post-fixative was used at a high ambient temperature (30°C) resulting in a fine precipitate of osmium decomposition products throughout the tissue. In addition, gross deposits of lead stain are present on the section.

should be carried out in a closed container in the presence of sodium hydroxide pellets. Full details of the method are given below.

We have found the most satisfactory staining procedure for renal biopsies to be a double staining technique using both uranium and lead. This produces more than double the contrast of either stain used alone and clearly delineates most tissue structures.

## VII. SECTION STAINING PROCEDURES

### A. Uranyl Acetate

*1. Saturated Uranyl Acetate in Methanol*

Saturate a small quantity (10 to 20 mℓ) of methanol with uranyl acetate. This may take several hours. Filter a little of the solution into a suitable container (e.g., a small petri dish) and immerse the grids to be stained. Close the container and protect from evaporation. A staining time of 20 to 30 min should be adequate. The grids are rinsed in three changes of 50% aqueous methanol at 30 to 40°C and allowed to dry.

*2. Saturated Uranyl Acetate in 70% Ethanol*

Saturate 10 to 20 mℓ of 70% aqueous ethanol with uranyl acetate. Filter a small amount of this solution and place drops of the filtrate onto a sheet of dental wax. The grids to be stained are floated on the drops for 20 to 30 min. The wax sheet should be

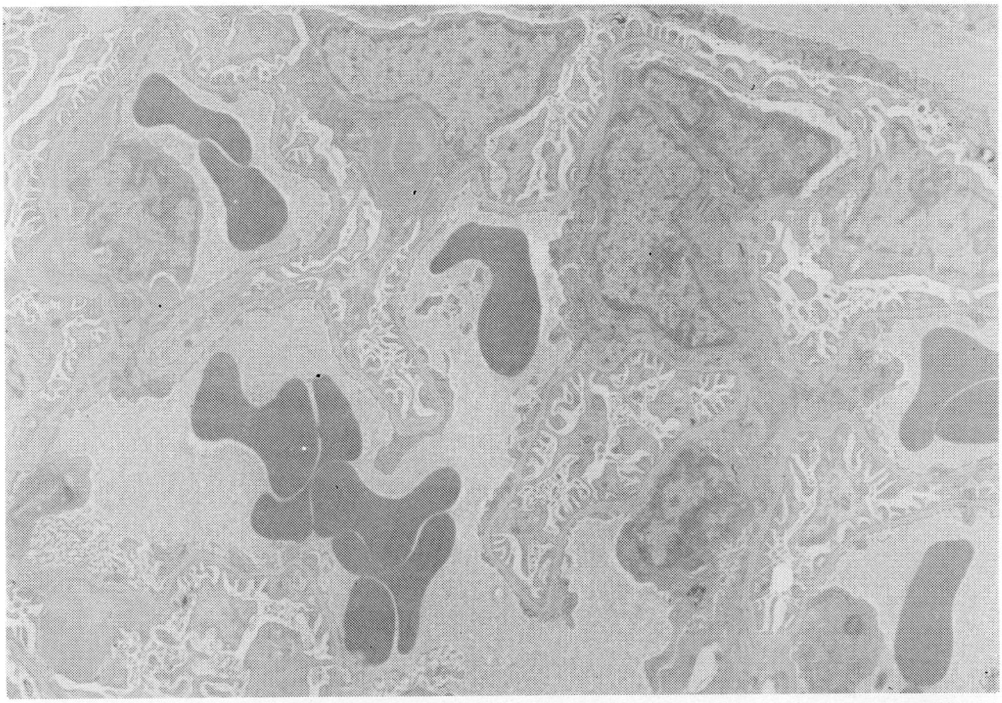

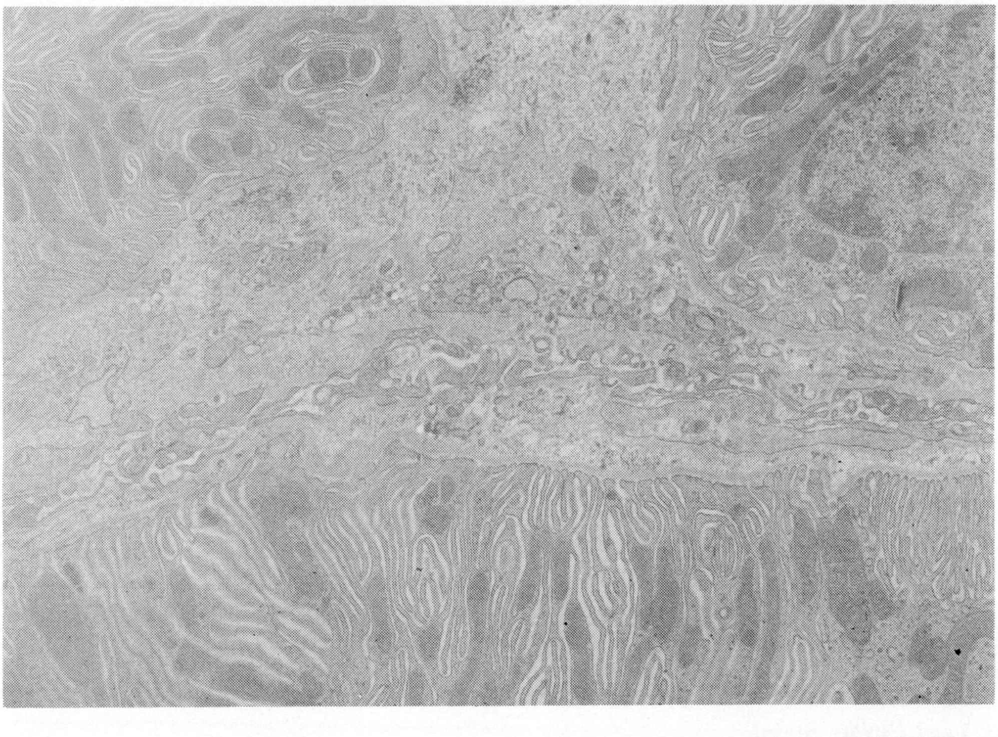

FIGURE 7 and 8. Rat kidney tissue. Fixation: PIPES buffered glutaraldehyde and paraformaldehyde. Staining: uranyl acetate in the block and uranyl acetate and lead citrate on the grid. (Magnification × 6800 for Figure 7 and × 15,000 for Figure 8, shown at 65%.) PIPES buffer results in minimal extraction. This results in micrographs of moderate contrast but showing considerable ultrastructural detail. Note the high density of mitochondria and other cytoplasmic features.

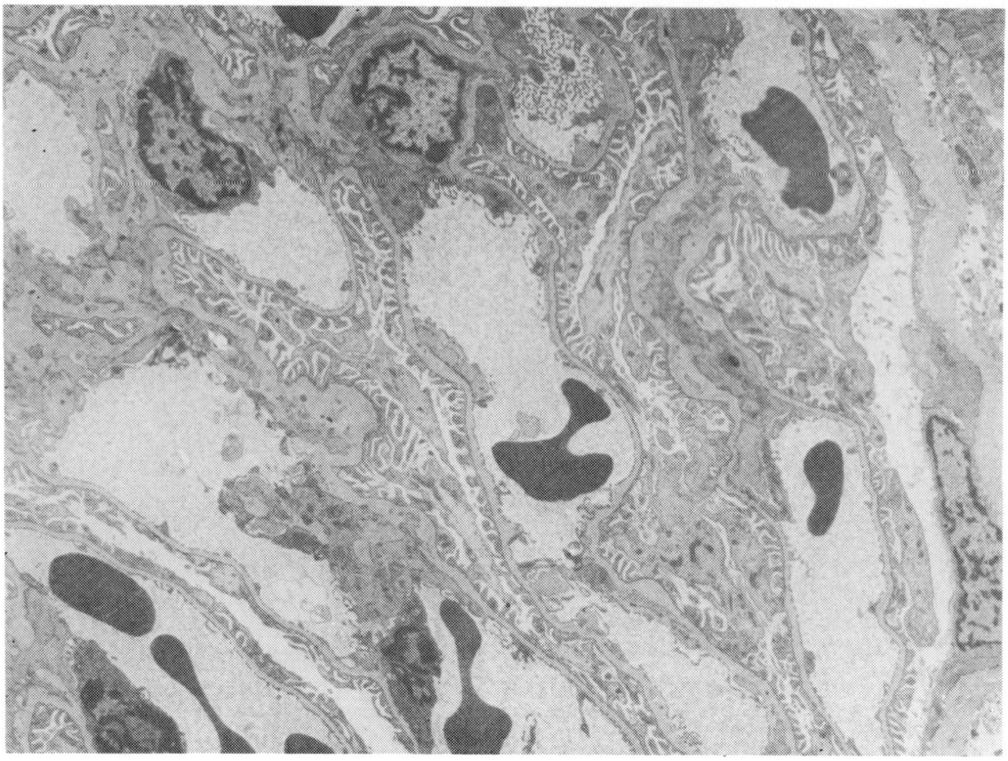

FIGURE 9. Rat kidney tissue. Fixation: Millonig's phosphate-buffered formalin, post-fixed in Dalton's fixative. Staining: uranyl acetate in the block and uranyl acetate and lead citrate on the grid. (Magnification × 6000 shown at 65%.) In comparison with Figures 7 and 8, there is increased extraction and some loss of detail. However, the results are suitable for diagnostic purposes. The extraction increases contrast between cellular features.

kept in a closed container during staining and it is advisable to include in the container a small, open petri dish containing 70% alcohol to decrease evaporation of the stain solvent. After staining, the grids are rinsed in one change of 70% ethanol and two changes of distilled water.

*3. Aqueous Uranyl Acetate*

Prepare a 5% solution of uranyl acetate by dissolving 2.5 g of the salt in 50 mℓ of distilled water. Grids are stained on drops of the filtered solution as above. Evaporation is much less of a problem with this method although a closed container should be used. Grids are rinsed in three changes of distilled water.

As solutions or uranyl acetate will undergo photodecomposition, it is advisable to store them in the dark. Staining operations should be protected from strong light sources. Uranyl acetate solutions should be discarded if they show signs of deposits or a change in color.

**B. Lead Citrate Stain**[13]

Weigh out 1.76 g of sodium citrate and 1.33 g of lead nitrate. Mix the solids and place in a 50-mℓ volumetric flask. Add approximately 30 mℓ of freshly boiled distilled water. Stopper the flask and shake vigorously for 2 min. Allow to stand with intermittent shaking for 30 min. Now add 8 mℓ of 1*M* sodium hydroxide (2 g/50 mℓ) and shake until the suspended solids dissolve. (Always use freshly prepared sodium hydroxide solution and protect from the air.) Finally, make up to 50 mℓ with freshly boiled distilled water.

Stain grid-mounted sections by floating the grids (section side down) on drops of the stain placed on strips of dental wax contained in a closed chamber containing sodium hydroxide pellets to absorb carbon dioxide. A staining time of 15 to 20 min is adequate. The sections are washed in three changes of freshly boiled distilled water.

The above techniques may be combined to yield additional contrast. Stain first with one of the uranyl acetate solutions; after washing, allow the sections to dry and then stain with the lead solution. The effects of this double staining process are shown in Figures 7 to 9.

### C. Permanganate Enhancement Technique

If still greater contrast is required, treatment of sections with buffered permanganate prior to the above double staining method will markedly increase contrast. This procedure is carried out as follows:

1. Immerse grid-mounted sections for 1 to 5 min on a freshly prepared 0.9% solution of potassium permanganate made up in 0.1 *M* phosphage buffer (pH 6.5) (see Chapter 2).
2. Wash for 2 min in 0.1 *M* phosphage buffer (pH 6.5).
3. Wash in 70% alcohol.
4. Double stain with uranyl acetate and lead citrate.[14]

It is occasionally desirable to use a more selective staining process to demonstrate with increased clarity such features as basement membrane changes or the deposition of immune complexes. In these cases the silver methenamine stain, originally developed for light microscopy, can be used to advantage. This procedure employs periodate oxidation to form aldehyde groups on carbonhydrate moities; these groups subsequently reduce the silver methenamine complex to electron opaque metallic silver. The method thus imparts considerable contrast to the glomerular basement membrane and other carbohydrate containing structures (e.g., glycogen). It was introduced as an EM stain by Marinozzi[15] and Movat[16] who applied the procedure to free-floating sections. Because of the number of reaction steps such a procedure is tedious. The staining reaction can be carried out with grid-mounted sections providing grids of an inert metal are used. Grids of gold, nickel, or stainless steel are suitable, with the latter being preferred for economy and ease of handling. The stain does not penetrate ARALDITE type resins and EPON is the recommended embedment. The silver methenamine stain is carried out as follows:

1. Oxidize the sections by immersing the grids in 1% periodic acid for 30 min at room temperature.
2. Wash thoroughly in distilled water (3 × 10 min).
3. Transfer to silver methenamine solution (Chapter 3) contained in a glass petri dish with a well-fitting lid. Place the dish in a 60°C incubator (in the dark). Staining is allowed to continue until the sections are a definite brown color. It is possible to wash a grid in distilled water, dry, and examine in the electron microscope and then replace it for further staining if the reaction has not proceeded far enough. However, with practice it is easy to determine when the reaction should be stopped from the color of the sections.
4. When staining is complete the grids are rinsed in several changes of distilled water and then allowed to dry. They are then ready for examination in the microscope (Figures 10 and 11).

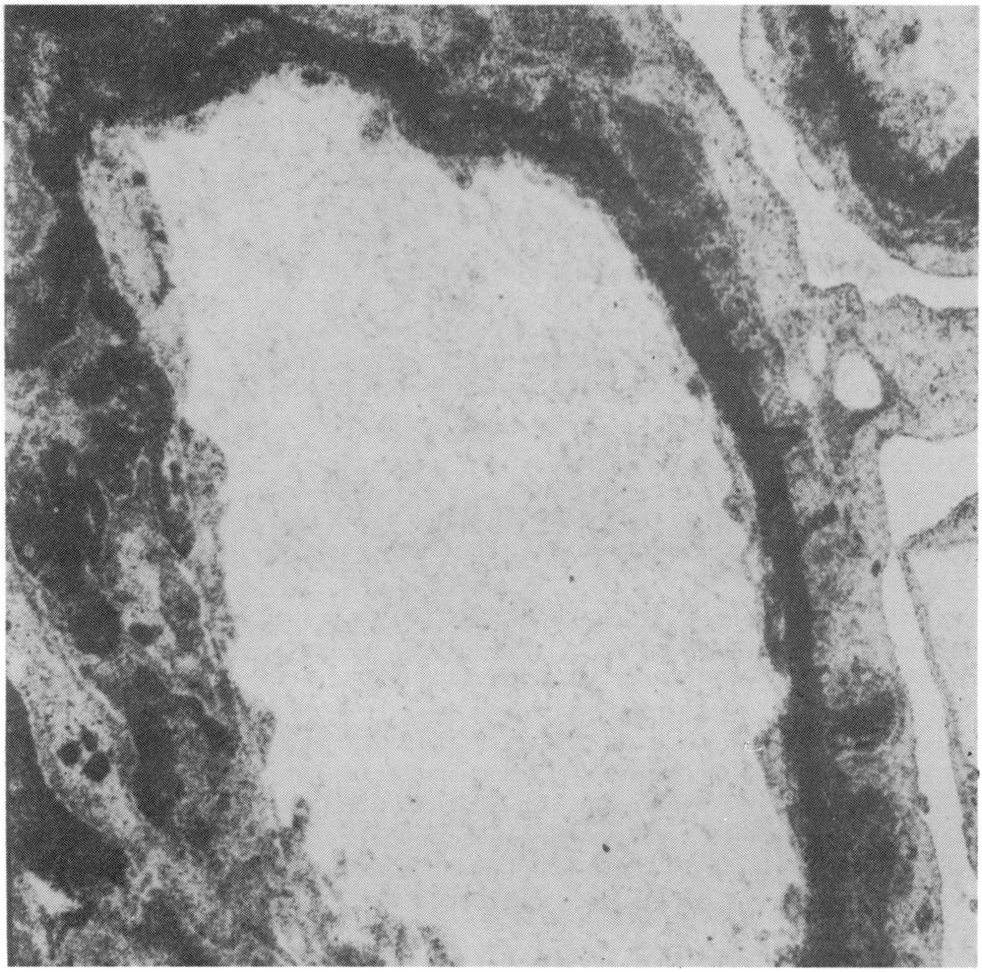

FIGURE 10. Early membranous glomerulonephritis with small argyrophilic epimembranous spikes and nonargyrophilic deposits. EPON embedment. Silver methenamine stain. (Magnification × 50,000.)

For EM it is even more important that only chemically clean glassware be used for the silver solution. Otherwise excessive random deposition of silver will occur, making the sections very messy. A good procedure is to reserve a new set of glassware for this stain and to keep this apparatus in a bath of 10% nitric acid when not in use. Prior to staining the acid is rinsed off with distilled water.

Although this staining reaction results in excellent contrast, it is only suitable for low- and moderate-power (up to × 10,000) micrographs. The grain structure of the silver deposit is rather coarse and this limits the resolution of the stain. We have tested an alternative method introduced by Thiery[17] in which thiocarbohydrazide is reacted with the aldehyde groups and the resulting combination is used to reduce silver proteinate to metallic silver. This sequence produces much smaller silver granules and, gives improved resolution but the degree of contrast is less as tissue components other than carbohydrates are stained. For this reason, we prefer the silver methenamine method for renal biopsy applications. Similar objections apply to the PATCO procedure of Hanker in which the aldehyde-thiocarbohydrazide combination is stained with oxmium tetroxide.[17] It is not-

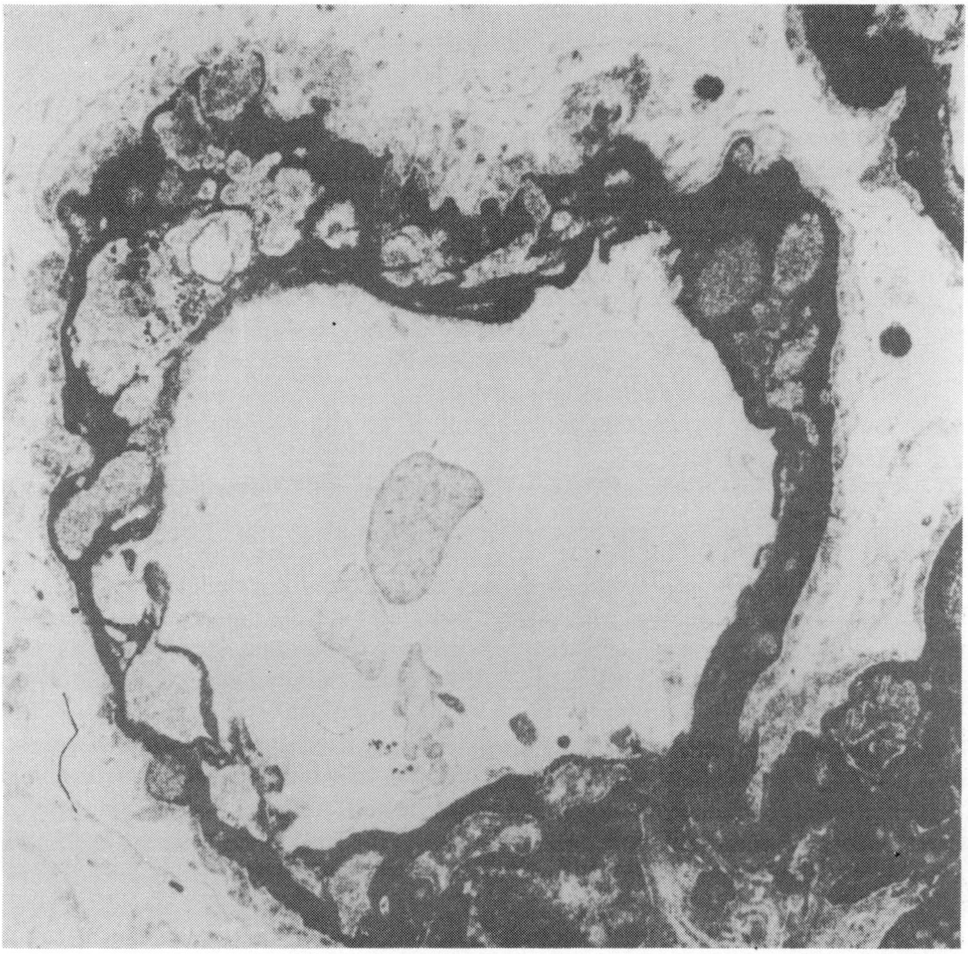

FIGURE 11. Advanced membranous nephropathy with spikes and "vacuoles" developing along the glomerular basement membrane. EPON embedment. Silver methenamine stain. (Magnification × 30,000.)

able that Cantin et al.[18] have reported successful staining of ARALDITE sections with Thiery's method.

### D. Alkaline Bismuth Method for Glycogen

The above method will stain glycogen granules. However, if the distribution of this material is of particular interest, a simpler and somewhat more selective stain may be used. The alkaline bismuth method of Ainsworth et al.[19] is suitable. In this method, tartrate-chelated bismuth ions are reduced to metallic bismuth by PAS-positive materials. In EPON sections glycogen is easily demonstrated by this method both with and without prior oxidation by periodate. Basement membranes are not stained, but there is some nonspecific staining of ribosomes and lysosomal-dense bodies. The stain is deposited as fine amorphous granules and the method is capable of high resolution. We have found the method to be unreliable if ARALDITE embedments are used.

#### *1. Method*

1. Cut ultrathin sections and mount on gold, nickel, or steel grids.

2. Float the grids, section side down, for 10 min at room temperature on buffered alcoholic periodic acid solution. This is prepared by dissolving 0.8 g of periodic acid in 70 mℓ of absolute alcohol then add 10 mℓ of M/5 sodium acetate and 20 mℓ of distilled water. This step may be omitted if desired as glycogen will stain without it although the reaction may be weaker.
3. Wash the sections by immersion in three changes of distilled water, 5 min each change.
4. Prepare an alkaline bismuth stock solution by dissolving 400 mg of potassium sodium tartrate in 10 mℓ of 2.0 *M* sodium hydroxide solution and adding this solution dropwise to 200 mg of bismuth subnitrate (oxynitrate), with constant stirring. The resulting solution should be clear. The staining solution is prepared by diluting 1 mℓ of the stock solution with 50 mℓ of distilled water. Both of these solutions will keep for one month at 4°C.
5. Float the grids, section side down, for 30 to 60 min at room temperature on the alkaline bismuth solution.
6. Rinse the grids briefly in 0.01 *M* sodium hydroxide solution and wash well in distilled water.

Ledingham and Simpson[20] applied an interesting staining technique to renal tissue. The tissue blocks were treated with phenylenediamine during dehydration. This simple method apparently produces contrast by reducing excess osmium residues in the tissue to "osmium blacks". The authors claim that this block stain produces sufficient contrast for light microscopy and low-power EM although additional staining with lead citrate is recommended for high-magnification work. We have tried this method and experienced some difficulty in obtaining uniform penetration of the stain. However, as staining is carried out during dehydration, the method may be useful in a rapid processing sequence and details are given below.

### E. Phenylenediamine Block Stain

Note that this method is applied to tissue blocks during dehydration and immediately following post-fixation with osmium tetroxide. It should not be applied to tissue treated with uranyl acetate.

1. Post-fix specimens in the usual manner (buffered osmium tetroxide or Dalton's fixative).
2. Rinse in 70% alcohol and transfer to 1% phenylenediamine (para isomer) in 70% alcohol for 30 min.
3. Rinse in 70% alcohol and continue the normal dehydration and embedding sequence.

According to the authors, 1 μm sections of tissue processed in this manner require no further staining for light microscopy and ultrathin sections need no other staining for low-power electron micrographs. **Caution:** p-Phenylenediamine can cause skin irritation and contact dermatitis. Handle with care and avoid breathing the dust.

## VIII. MICROSCOPY AND PHOTOGRAPHY

The results of the electron microscopic examination of biopsies will invariably be recorded on photographic film. It is impractical for the microscopist to attempt to remember the features of any particular biopsy and only a photograph can completely record the information present in the electron image. All electron microscopes are equipped with photographic facilities and the details of operation of these will be covered in the manufacturer's handbook. Older machines were equipped only with plate cameras and while these can produce micrographs of the highest quality, glass plates are easily damaged and, because of their fragility, size, and weight, they are difficult to store. More recently the trend has been to include roll or sheet film facilities. Often the older plate cameras can be adapted to take sheet film. This change is recommended since the sheets are far easier to handle and the marginal reduction in dimensional stability only has significance in very high-resolution microscopy. Where suitable cameras can be fitted to the microscope, roll film is by far the most convenient photographic format for biopsy work. Apart from the ease of handling, it offers a large number of exposures at one loading. This feature is often useful since "difficult" biopsies may require the examination and discussion of many areas to arrive at a diagnosis. Objections to the use of roll film have included difficulties in degassing the film prior to loading in the microscope and problems of static discharges exposing the film as it is transported through the camera mechanism. Provided a supply of film is kept in a vacuum desiccator, the first objection is overcome and modern camera designs have largely eliminated the second problem. Two-roll film formats are found in EM cameras, 35 and 70 mm. We favor the smaller format since it offers considerable savings in materials costs and the image quality is more than adequate. A 35-mm camera will usually cover a larger image area than any of the other formats although at a magnification somewhat less than that attained on the viewing screen. This situation arises since the 35-mm camera is frequently positioned in the microscope column, below the projector lens, and above the final screen. Supplies of 35-mm film are generally easier to obtain than are 70-mm rolls and the narrower film seems to suffer less from "in camera" transport problems.

Prior to loading photographic materials into the microscope it is important that they be degassed in a vacuum desiccator. Films and plates stored under normal atmospheric conditions absorb appreciable quantities of water vapor and this, together with plasticizer vapors from sheet and roll film, will be evolved when the film is placed in the vacuum of the microscope. These vapors will contaminate the vacuum system, resulting in long pumping times and ultimately in a degradation of image quality through specimen contamination. Many microscopes incorporate a vacuum desiccator for this purpose, but a separate vacuum tank coupled to a rotary pump is preferable. In the former arrangement gasses from the film still contaminate the microscope pump. If the microscope pump must be used, careful attention should be paid to venting the pump oil at regular intervals by operating the pump in the "gas-ballast" mode. Oil changes may also have to be made more frequently. Separate desiccators are available from a number of manufacturers (see Appendix).

A tray containing phosphorous pentoxide is usually kept in the vacuum chamber to absorb displaced moisture. This material absorbs water vapor more effectively than any other drying agent, but must be used with care. The powder reacts explosively with water producing toxic choking fumes, and the resulting mixture is very corrosive (phosphoric acid). The powdered oxide should not be allowed to blow onto film or film containers or into the rotary pump. As it absorbs moisture a sticky film will form over the oxide and this must be removed at frequent intervals to expose fresh oxide layers. Never attempt to dissolve the layer with water as underlying oxide may well cause an explosion. Small pieces of the layer can be stripped off with a spatula and added to a large volume of water, preferably in a fume cupboard. It is possible to purchase phosphorous pentoxide absorbed onto an inert substrate (Merck); this is claimed to overcome the need to remove spent oxide at intervals.

A loaded Philips® 35-mm film cassette requires 6 to 8 hr in a desiccator at −100 kPa and containing fresh phosphorous pentoxide for adequate degassing. Normally, cassettes are placed in the vacuum chamber at least 24 hr before use and we have experienced no problems with film that has been dried for over a week. Sheet films and plates can be expected to degas more rapidly than 35-mm rolls while 70-mm rolls would require longer. Film should be transferred from desiccator to microscope vacuum as rapidly as possible to prevent the reabsorption of moisture.

The adjustment and operation of the microscope to produce a correctly exposed negative should be adequately described in the manufacturer's handbook. These instructions should be followed carefully and every effort made to achieve correct exposure. The correction of errors at a later processing stage will be time consuming and correction processes will never produce a result as good as that given by a properly formed negative. In particular, the microscope should be properly aligned, lens astigmatism corrected, and the illumination adjusted to evenly cover the screen and provide a reasonable exposure time. This will usually be of the order of 1 to 2 sec. Shorter exposures may result in radiation damage to the specimen while longer times can produce blurred images from vibration. Some form of exposure meter is essential for reproducible results. Many microscopes now include such devices which function by measuring the radiation density on the microscope screen. Alternatively, a photometer may be used to measure the light intensity emitted by the final screen.

Where fitted, it is recommended that specimen anticontamination devices be used. These enable specimens to be examined for long periods of time without noticeable deterioration. In biopsy work, much time is frequently spent examining small areas of the specimen before a photograph is taken.

The contrast of the microscope image is commonly varied to suit individual preference by adjusting the section staining times. However, it should be borne in mind that contrast may also be adjusted by using the microscope controls. An increase of accelerating voltage will decrease contrast and give increased image brightness and increased resolution. This is often useful when examining a thick section. Conversely, lower accelerating voltages will give somewhat lower resolution and decreased brightness but more contrast. Many microscopists choose to work at 60 kV although in fact generally better results can be obtained at higher voltages. These factors should not be used as an excuse for the use of thicker sections.

Contrast is also influenced by the size of the objective aperture fitted to the microscope. In general, the smaller the aperture, the greater the contrast. A common aperture size in 50 $\mu$m and a considerable increase in contrast will be noticed if this is reduced to 30 or 20$\mu$m. However, the smaller apertures will reduce the image brightness and be more prone to contamination. The contamination problem is reduced if "thin foil" apertures are used which are to some extent self-cleaning, but frequent checks of the objective system astigmatism should still be made.

The sequence of events for recording the microscope image on film is as follows:

1. Select an area of the specimen of interest and place in the center of the screen. Bring into approximate focus with the microscope controls.
2. Adjust the magnification of the microscope so that the area of interest is within the screen area that appears on the negative. (This area is usually marked on the screen.)
3. Adjust the focusing binoculars to suit the operator's eyes and then accurately focus the microscope image. Some microscopes have "wobbler" focusing aids to facilitate this process.
4. Adjust the microscope illumination to a level appropriate for photography; usually a reference level is provided by an exposure meter. Ensure that the illumination is evenly distributed across the screen.
5. Make the exposure and record the details of the photograph on a record sheet.

## Table 2
## SOME KODAK® FILMS FOR ELECTRON MICROSCOPY[21]

| Material[a] | Recommended development[b] | Safelight | Size |
|---|---|---|---|
| | at 68°F (20°C) with continuous agitation | | |
| Electron image plate | Maximum speed D. 19 12 min | No. 1 | 6.5 × 9.0 cm |
| | HRP (1:2) 5 min | | 3¼ × 4 in. |
| | | | 3¼ × 3¼ in. |
| | Intermediate speed | | |
| | D. 19 (1:2) 4 min | | |
| | plus Ig/L anti-fog No. 1 | | |
| | HRP (1:4) 3 min | | |
| | plus Ig/L anti-fog No. 1 | | |
| | Minimum Grain D. 19 2 min | | |
| | plus Ig/L anti-fog No. 1 | | |
| | HRP (1:4) 3 min | | |
| Electron microscope film | D. 19 (1:2) 4 min | No. 1A | 2 × 10 in. |
| | | OA | 3¼ × 4 in. |
| | | OC | 3¼ × 3 5/16 in. |
| | | | 6.5 × 9.0 cm |
| | | | 7 × 7 cm |
| Kodalith® LR film | D. 19 2 min | No. 1A | 35 mm × 150 ft |
| Type 2572 (estar base) | D. 19 (1:2) 4 min | | 70 mm × 150 ft |
| Eastman fine grain release | D. 19 2 min | No. OA | 35 mm × 100 ft |
| Positive film type 5302 | D. 19 (1:2) 4 min | | 70 mm × 100 ft |
| | Dektol 2 min | | |

[a] Estar base materials pump down more quickly than those with an acetate base.
[b] Longer development enables better control.

The following notes may aid the production of quality negatives. It is generally preferable to take photographs at the lowest useful magnification. Critical focusing is then easier and more likely to be accurate and further magnification will be introduced when the negative is printed. This additional optical magnification can be up to 6 to 8× without noticeable deterioration of the image. There should not be an extreme difference between the illumination level at which fine focusing is carried out and that at which the photograph is taken. A drastic change in illumination is often accompanied by specimen movement due to changes in the heating effect of the electron beam. These effects are magnified near holes or other areas of physical weakness in the specimen. If possible, photographs should be taken of areas away from such defects. It is vital that records be kept of the photographs taken. Every film or plate should be numbered and such details as the name or code number of the specimen should be recorded. It is often a help to briefly describe the area photographed or the item of interest. Some workers prefer to make a rough sketch or diagram on the record sheet. This can provide a useful memory aid to the relevance of the photograph.

If there is any doubt over the relevance or importance of any feature seen in the biopsy specimen, it should be photographed. Film and photographic facilities are inexpensive compared with the other processes involved in EM and it can be surprisingly difficult to again find an item previously left unrecorded.

The processing of photographic material from the microscope will depend on the type of film being used. Table 2 lists film types supplied by Kodak® for EM together with the recommended developers. Film from other manufacturers is usually similar to one of the Kodak® products and can be processed in a similar manner.

In some countries it is occasionally difficult to obtain supplies of the specialist films for EM, or there may be a large minimum order requirement. In such situations we have obtained excellent results from Kodak® Graphic Arts Film (Kodak® Ortho Film, Type 3, Code 2256.) This film has a thin, high-contrast, blue-sensitive emulsion coated onto a thin estar base. This material is readily available due to its wide use in various graphic reproduction processes. Unfortunately, the film is not marketed in standard EM sizes, but it can be purchased as 8- × 10-in. sheets. These are easily cut to the required size as the film can be handled under the usual safelights. The main disadvantage of this film is its slow electron film speed. It requires approximately 10 times the exposure of the normal film types. Development is in D19 using the conditions given below for film type 5302. (Exposure time may be decreased by extending development time.)

**A. Photographic Processing**

Full details of recommended processing methods are always available from the film manufacturer. However, many microscopists prefer to develop their own films at least to the negative stage as the process is reasonably simple and allows rapid assessment of the success (or otherwise) of a microscope session. For this reason the necessary processing details are given below.

Most commonly, film or plates will be processed to a negative which is subsequently used to prepare a print on photographic paper. Printing techniques are more specialized and outside the scope of this book, but a full description can be found in many photographic manuals. As an alternative to printing, it is possible to reverse process films and plates to produce positive transparencies. This technique is particularly useful when 35-mm roll film is used in the microscope as slides for projection at seminars, etc. are then readily produced. The technique produces slides having very fine grain and, if necessary, a negative can be produced at a later stage by a standard film copying process. The contrast of the slides produced in this manner is controlled by the contrast on the microscope image.

Positive transparencies may also be produced by copying negatives onto a suitable copying film (e.g., see Kodak® book for details). Frequently a better result is produced by rephotographing a carefully produced print, the camera film then being reversed processed to give a slide. With this method marks or scratches on the negative can be retouched on the print and magnification markers can be included if necessary. Also, it is easy to be selective of the areas being rephotographed. A fine grain film such as Panatomic® X can produce very good slides in this manner. Particularly good results are obtained if a color reversal film (e.g., Ektachrome®) is used for the rephotography. Although using a color film to produce a black and white image may seem uneconomical, the results are aesthetically satisfying. A very dense black is produced by color film and the rest of the gray scale has a pleasing tone.

**B. Correction of Over- or Underexposed Film**

It is inevitable that an occasional negative or slide will turn out to be over- or underexposed. For this reason an intensifier and a reducing formula are given below. These solutions should only be used on negatives when the original is unusable and cannot be repeated. The grain structure of the negative is adversely affected by both intensification and reduction, and subsequent prints will never approach the quality obtainable from a good negative. The solutions are of more use when the microscope film is reverse processed to slides. Here, the effects on the grain structure of moderate intensification or reduction are not noticeable. In particular, when there is some doubt as to the quality of the microscope image we have found it preferable to produce over-dense slides and then correct them to optimum appearance with reducer. This process can be done with individual frames if necessary.

Whatever the form of photographic record used it is important that the processing be carried out carefully to ensure permanence. Any tendency to shorten fixing and washing times should be resisted since improperly fixed or washed films and prints will eventually discolor. Negatives, prints, and slides should be adequately labeled and stored away from light in a place not subject to high temperatures or humidity as these factors will encourage the growth of mold and accelerate deterioration. Storage cabinets should be of robust construction since in many cases the photographic record will be the only record of the biopsy. In some renal conditions other areas of the biopsy may not show the same features and so resectioning may not be possible.

## IX. PHOTOGRAPHIC PROCESSING

Plates and sheet film are best placed in racks and developed in tanks. Alternatively, they may be developed in dishes under the recommended safelight conditions. Roll film is fed into a spiral for tank development. A typical processing sequence is given below (for 35-mm film). Precise development conditions for any particular film are usually included in the film packaging or are readily available from the manufacturer.

### A. Negative Development Procedure for Kodak® 35-mm Film Type 5302

1. Load film under recommended safelight conditions (type OA).
2. Add sufficient developer to fill tank to the recommended level (Kodak® D 19 diluted 1:2 at 20°C).
3. Invert tank continuously for the first 15 sec then once every 30 sec. Total development time is 4 min. Discard the developer.
4. Quickly wash the film with running water, changing the contents of the tank at least three times.
5. Fill the tank with fixer (e.g., Kodafix®), agitate frequently for a total of 4 min.
6. Wash the film in running water for 10 min.
7. Rinse with photo-flo solution at the recommended dilution. Steps 6 and 7 are conveniently done with the film still in the tank.
8. Remove the film from the tank and dry in a warm dust-free area.

### B. Reverse Processing Sequence for the Production of Positive Transparencies

*1. Solutions*

Tap water, filtered if necessary, should be used for these solutions as distilled water is too soft and may cause reticulation.

#### *a. Bleach Stock Solution*

| | |
|---|---|
| Sodium dichromate | 40 g |
| Concentrated Sulfuric acid | 50 mℓ |
| Water to 1 ℓ | |

Dissolve the chromate in the water and then *slowly* add the acid with stirring. For use dilute this stock 1 + 9 with water.

#### *b. Clear Solution*

| | |
|---|---|
| Sodium sulfite (anhydrous) | 100 g |
| Sodium hydroxide | 2 g |
| Water to 2 ℓ | |

Mix the sulfite with a little water for form a slurry. Add this to the remaining water with stirring. Finally, add and dissolve the sodium hydroxide. If the sulfite is not slurried first, it will hydrate to a hard lump which is very difficult to dissolve.

***c. Developers***

**First developer (for Kodak® films)** — Kodak® D19 with the addition of 2.2g/ℓ sodium thiocyanate ($2H_2O$).

**Second developer** — Kodak® D19.

**Fixer** — Any hardening fixer.

*2. Processing Method*

| | |
|---|---|
| First Develop | 7 min at 20°C<br>Agitate continuously for 15 sec then invert the tank once every 30 sec, this time is suitable for Kodak® 35-mm film type 5302; the optimum time for other film types should be determined from a test strip |
| Wash | 3 min in running water |
| Bleach | 3 min continuous agitation |
| Wash | 3 min running water |
| Clear | 3 min continuous agitation |
| Wash | 3 min running water |
| Fog | Either remove the film from the spiral and expose each side to a 60-W lamp at a distance of 1 ft. for 1½ to 2 min or if spiral is translucent, expose each side to lamp for 3 min |
| Second develop | 3 min with continuous agitation |
| Wash | 3 min in running water |
| Fix | 3 min continuous agitation |
| Wash running water for 10 min | |

Finally, treat the film briefly with a solution of wetting agent (e.g., photoflo) and remove from reel and hang to dry in a dust free area. The dry film can then be cut into individual frames and mounted into slide holders. There are numerous types of these available from photographic dealers. For the Philips® EM format 126 size slide holders are suitable.

**C. Reducing and Intensifying Solutions**

These solutions are applied to fully processed and washed negatives or slides.

*1. Farmers Reducer*

This solution may be used for reducing the density of overexposed and overdeveloped slides and negative. Note, however, that overexposed negatives will generally have excessive contrast as well as excessive density and reduction will tend to emphasize grain structure. The solution is particularly useful for the reduction of slides produced by the reversal process. (see Section IX.B).

| | |
|---|---|
| Solution A | 37.5 g |
| Potassium ferricyanide | |
| Water to 500 mℓ | |
| Solution B | 480 g |
| Sodium thiosulfate | |
| Water to 2 ℓ | |

For use mix 1 part of Solution A with 4 parts of Solution B and add 27 parts of water. The overdense negative or slide should be thoroughly wetted and it is then treated with the reducer until a satisfactory density remains. Wash thoroughly after treatment and dry in the usual manner.

### B. Intensifier Solution

This solution may also be used on both slides and negatives, but again an increase in granularity may be noticed when the intensified negative is printed. Moderate intensification is hardly noticeable on slides. The following solutions must be made up in distilled water:

| | |
|---|---|
| A. Silver nitrate | 60 g |
| Distilled water to 1ℓ | |
| B. Sodium sulfite (anhydrous) | 60 g |
| Distilled water to 1ℓ | |
| C. Sodium thiosulfate | 105 g |
| Distilled water to 1ℓ | |
| D. Elon (p-methylaminophenol sulfate) | 25 g |
| Sodium sulfite | |
| Distilled water to 3ℓ | |

These solutions do not keep well so only prepare an amount that can be used in 1 to 2 weeks.

Ensure that the slide or negative is thoroughly wet and give a final rinse in distilled water. To prepare the intensifier solution for use slowly add one part of Solution B to one part of Solution A and mix thoroughly. Dissolve the white precipitate by the addition of one part of Solution C. Allow the resulting solution to stand a few minutes until clear. Then add while stirring three parts of Solution D. The film should be treated immediately with this mixture. The degree of intensification depends on the time of treatment which should not exceed 25 min. After intensification refix the film in a 30% sodium thiosulfate solution. All dishes used for these solutions must be chemically clean and the operations should be carried out in artificial light. Further details of these reducing and intensifying solutions may be found in the Kodak® data book.[22]

## X. SPECIAL METHODS — PREPARATION FOR EM OF MATERIAL PROCESSED FOR OPTICAL MICROSCOPY

### A. Plastic-Embedded Specimens

Ultrathin sections for EM may be cut directly from these blocks after they have been trimmed to isolate the area of interest. The sections are collected, stained, and examined in the usual way. The results given by this process are rather poor in terms of ultrastructural preservation, but they can be diagnostically useful. Basement membrane material is usually quite well preserved and the additional resolution of the electron microscope can aid diagnosis in difficult situations (Figure 12).

### B. Paraffin-Embedded Specimens

The area of interest in the biopsy is carefully cut out of the paraffin block using a warm razor blade. It is then treated as follows:

1. Place in excess xylene (×10) until the residual wax has dissolved.
2. Wash for 10 min in each of two changes of xylene.
3. Wash in graded alcohols (abs; 90%; 70%; 50%) 5 min in each.
4. Wash in water or in buffer (0.1 *M* cacodylate PIPES or phosphate pH. 7.4).

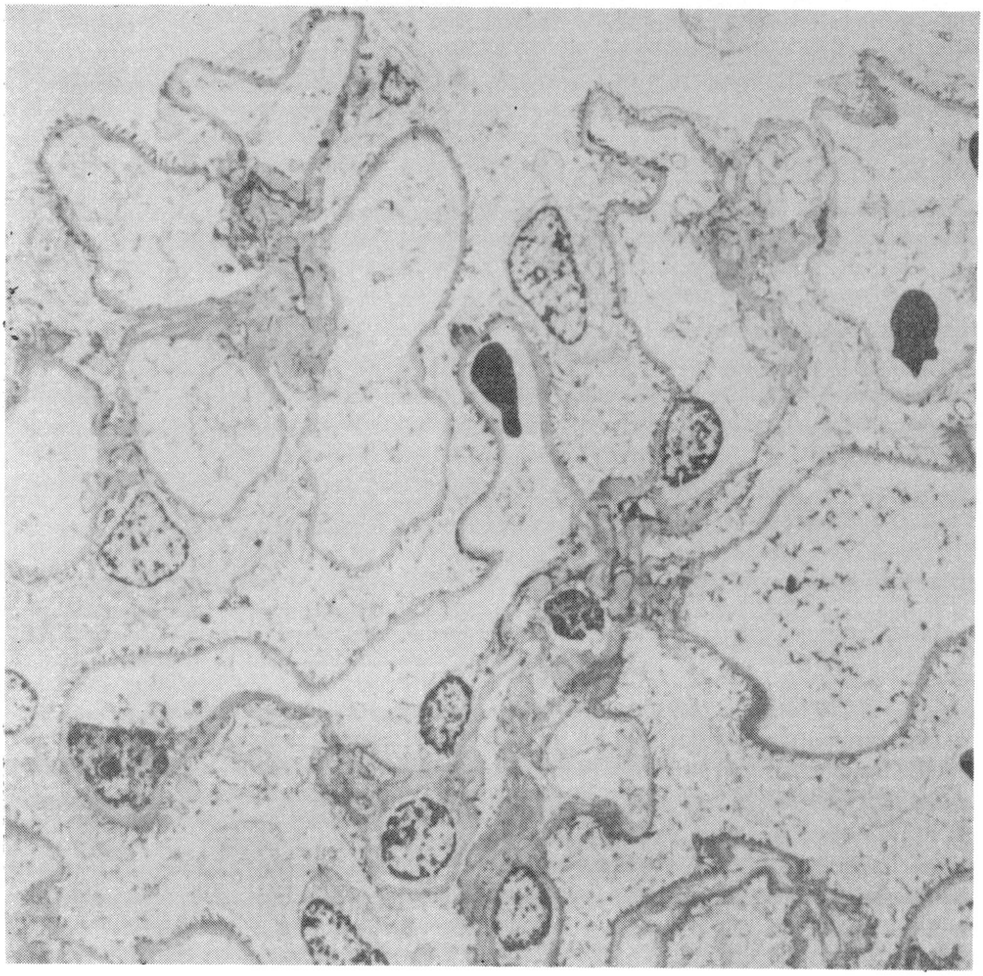

FIGURE 12. Electron micrograph of glomerulus following Duboscq-Brasil fixation and embedment in Spurrs resin. Staining: uranyl acetate and lead citrate on the grid. (Magnification × 3300.)

5. Post-fix in 1% osmium tetroxide in water or buffer for 1 hr.
6. Wash in buffer and dehydrate and embed in epoxy resin as described in Section III.C.

The embedded specimen is then sectioned, stained, and examined in the normal way. Results are generally rather poor with considerable shrinkage and extraction of cellular components. Again, however, they may provide useful information in difficult cases (Figure 12).

## REFERENCES

1. **Glauert, A. M.,** Fixation, dehydration and embedding of biological specimens, in *Practical Methods in Electron Microscopy,* Vol. 3 (Part 1), Glauert, Ed., North-Holland, Amsterdam, 1975.
2. **Mollenhauer, H. H.,** Plastic embedding mixtures for use in electron microscopy , *Stain Technol.,* 39, 111, 1964.
3. **Dettman, H. and Pearson, C. B.,** Better epoxy resin embedding for electron microscopy at low relative humidity, *Stain Technol.,* 52, 5, 1977.

4. **Muller, L. L. and Jacks, T. J.,** Rapid chemical dehydration of samples for electron microscopic examinations, *J. Histochem. Cytochem.,* 23, 107, 1975.
5. **McNelly, N. and Hinds, J.,** Rescuing poorly embedded tissue for EM. A new and simple technique on re-embedding, *Stain Technol.,* 50, 209, 1975.
6. **Reid, N.,** Ultramicrotomy, in *Practical Methods in Electron Microscopy,* Vol. 3 (Part 2), Glauert, Ed., North-Holland, Amsterdam, 1975.
7. **Richardson, K. C., Jarett, L., and Finke, E. H.,** Embedding in epoxy resins for ultrathin sectioning in EM, *Stain Technol.,* 35, 313, 1960.
8. **Lee, J. C. and Hooper, J., Jr.,** Basic fuchsin-crystal violet: a rapid staining sequence for juxtaglomerular granules embedded in epoxy resin, *Stain Technol.,* 40, 37, 1965.
9. **Yang, G. and Morrison, A.,** Wide field electron microscopy, *Am. J. Clin. Pathol.,* 64, 648, 1975.
10. **Lewis, P. R. and Knight, D. P .,** Staining methods for sectioned material, in *Practical Methods in Electron Microscopy,* Vol. 5 (Part 1), Glauert, Ed., North-Holland, Amsterdam, 1977.
11. **Allen, D. E. and Perrin, D. D.,** Electron cytochemical stains based on metal chelation, *Int. Rev. Cytol.,* 61, 63, 1979.
12. **Hayat, M. A.,** Biological applications, in *Principles and Techniques of Electron Microscopy,* Vol. 1, Van Nostrand Reinhold, New York, 1970, 253.
13. **Reynolds, E. S.,** The use of lead citrate at high pH as an electron opaque stain in electron microscopy, *J. Cell Biol.,* 17, 208, 1963.
14. **Lewis, P. R. and Knight, D. P.,** Staining methods for sectioned material, in *Practical Methods in Electron Microscopy,* Vol. 5 (Part 1), Glauert, Ed., North-Holland, Amsterdam, 1977, 59.
15. **Marinozzi, V.,** Silver impregnation of ultrathin sections for electron microscopy, *J. Biophys. Biochem. Cytol.,* 9, 121, 1961.
16. **Movat, H. Z.,** Silver impregnation methods for electron microscopy, *Am. J. Clin. Pathol.,* 35, 528, 1961.
17. **Thiery, J. P.,** Mise en evidence des polysaccharides sur coupes fines en microscopie electronique, *J. Microscopie,* 6, 987, 1967.
18. **Cantin, M., Desormeaux, Y., Chlebovicova, J., Benchimol, S., and de Aravjo-Nascimento, M.,** Comparative ultrastructural cytochemistry of juxtaglomerular cell granules and renal tubular cell lysosomes, *Lab. Invest.,* 33, 648, 1975.
19. **Ainswonth, S. K., Ito, S., and Karnovsky, M. J.,** Alkaline bismuth reagent for high resolution ultrastructural demonstration of periodate reactive sites, *J. Histochem. Cytochem.,* 20, 995, 1972.
20. **Ledingham, J. M. and Simpson, F. O.,** The use of p-phenylenediamine in the block to enhance osmium staining for electron microscopy, *Stain Technol.,* 47, 239, 1972.
21. **Kodak,** *Electron Microscopy and Photography,* Eastman Kodak, Rochester, 1973.
22. *Kodak Data Book,* Section FY5, Kodak, London, 1973, 3 and 7.

Chapter 5

# THE CLINICAL RELEVANCE OF METHODS SELECTED FOR OPTICAL AND ELECTRON MICROSCOPY

**David E. Allen and John P. Dowling**

## TABLE OF CONTENTS



## I. INTRODUCTION

In general, staining procedures are selected to highlight tissue components that have undergone pathological change. The light microscopic definition of renal pathology requires the demonstration of such tissue components as basement membrane (glomerular and tubular), mesangial matrix, glomerular cells, deposited protein, inflammatory cells, tubular cell cytoplasm, vessels, and the accumulation of substances such as amyloid, calcium salts, and various pigments.

It has become apparent from our own experience and that of others that there is considerable variation in the ability of different staining methods to demonstrate these elements, particularly in relation to the use of different fixatives and embedding media.

## II. HEMATOXYLIN AND EOSIN

The traditional H & E remains an excellent all-purpose stain regardless of the fixative or embedding medium used. Careful inspection of the H- & E-stained renal biopsy will often reveal the presence of changes such as glomerular protein deposits, glomerular basement membrane, and general cytoplasmic alteration. It remains as the best general stain for distinguishing the different types of inflammatory cells infiltrating the kidney. Hematoxylin identifies the abnormal nuclear masses seen in the renal involvement of systemic lupus erythaematosus, namely the hematoxyphil bodies[1] and calcium deposits are usually intensely hematoxyphilic. By contrast, eosin demonstrates the inclusion bodies seen in such viral infections as herpes simplex and cytomegalovirus.

In paraffin sections, the eosinophilia of glomerular basement membrane, mesangial matrix, and mesangial cell cytoplasm prevents a distinction between the structures. In contrast in plastic-embedded material, the refractile pale staining of the matrix and basement membrane differentiates these structures from mesangial cell cytoplasm. An alternative cytoplasmic stain is phloxine. This is particularly useful in demonstrating intracellular inclusions.

## III. PERIODIC ACID-SCHIFF'S (PAS) REACTION

This widely applied stain accentuates basement membrane structures because of its affinity for carbohydrate moities[2] (Plate 1).* It often provides the sharpest outline of arteriolar and arterial hyalinosis. Hyalin, composed partly of plasma proteins stains intensely in the PAS reaction.[3] The "sludgy" deposits seen in the paraproteinaemic glomerulonephropathies are often PAS positive.[4] Tamm-Horsfall protein, possibly an important cause of interstitial damage is also PAS positive.[5]

This staining method is seen to best advantage in paraffin sections irrespective of the fixation used. In resin sections we have experienced some variability in staining and, on occasions, noted the persistence of a fine, artifactual granularity in some areas of the section.

## IV. MASSON'S TRICHROME

With protracted use, we have found the Masson's trichrome to be a reliable and sensitive indicator of glomerular deposits, basement membrane changes, cytoplasmic alterations, and the degree of glomerular and interstitial "scarring". Duboscq-Brasil fixative has provided a better demonstration particularly of glomerular protein deposits than other fixatives in biopsies embedded both in paraffin and resin. We agree with Cohen[6] that it is both an accurate and inexpensive means of defining renal pathology and that with the finding of often minute glomerular protein deposits EM may prove unnecessary.

The red mixture selected for the protein stain in this method is stronger than those usually used. This stronger mixture has consistently improved the localization of protein deposits in renal tissue with good correlation between the Masson stain, immunohistochemistry, and EM.

* Plate 1 appears following page 88.

## V. SILVER METHENAMINE

The periodic acid silver methenamine stain is now accepted as one which produces in both paraffin and plastic-embedded renal tissue the clearest outline of the glomerular basement membrane, the mesangium and tubular basement membranes, and of changes related to these structures. Since its description by Jones in 1957,[7] this method has been responsible for delineating many of the basic structural changes that occur, particularly in glomerulonephritis. Precise definition of the glomerular basement membrane, especially in sections cut at 2 $\mu$m or less can demonstrate subtle or early lesions such as fine localized epimembranous "spike" formation in membranous glomerulonephritis or lamellation of capillary loops in Alport's syndrome. In this respect, resin-embedded sections, by producing thinner sections, show a clear-cut advantage over paraffin.

The silver methenamine stain may be applied either alone or in combination with several counterstains. Without counterstains, the altered structures are thrown into stark relief. Combination with hematoxylin and eosin allows one to assess cellular detail more accurately, but in some cases the silver-impregnated components appear too heavily stained if Harris' or Weigert's hematoxylin is used; lighter staining is achieved with Carazzi's hematoxylin combined with eosin.

## VI. SILVER METHENAMINE-TRICHROME

We are indebted to Burkholder[8] who, in his *Atlas of Human Glomerular Pathology,* outlined his method for a combined silver methenamine and Masson's trichrome staining procedure. With Duboscq-Brasil fixation, this technique has provided excellent results in both paraffin- and plastic-embedded sections. Good contrast is achieved between the basement membrane, mesangial matrix, cell cytoplasm, and protein deposits (Plates 2 and 3).* It has often been noted that the latter are more clearly outlined with better contrast by the Masson stain in combination with the silver than with the trichrome alone. For photographic purposes particularly, this combination often provides a beautiful demonstration of the lesions present. In this regard, the use of the fast green stain in the Masson's trichrome appears to give clearer contrast than aniline blue. To emphasize, we believe this combined staining method greatly facilitates diagnosis in nephropathology.

## VII. SILVER METHENAMINE-CHROMOTROPE 2R

This stain was applied by Ehrenreich and Espinosa[9] to renal biopsies fixed in neutral 10% formalin or Bouin's fluid and embedded in paraffin. We have also found it to be a reliable method of demonstrating both basement membrane changes and the presence of small and large protein deposits in tissue fixed in Duboscq-Brasil fixative and embedded in paraffin. Similarly, fixed resin embedded sections provided less reliable staining of the deposits by the chromotrope 2R.

## VIII. MARTIUS SCARLET BLUE

Since 1962[10] this trichrome stain has been used to demonstrate the presence of "fibrinoid" (fibrin and other plasma proteins) within the kidney and many other tissues. After some years of use it appears to be less specific for fibrin than originally claimed. However, this stain does differentiate between old and more recent hyalin deposits in

* Plates 2 and 3 appear following page 88.

renal tissues, particularly when the tissue is mordanted prior to staining. In this instance, glutaraldehyde fixation has the advantage of delineating fine glomerular immune-complex deposits seen in glomerulonephritis. This remains true for both paraffin embedded and resin embedded biopsies. Fixation solely in Duboscq-Brasil solution does not result in optimal staining with this technique.

## IX. ELASTIN STAINS

Vascular pathology is an important facet of nephropathology and a clear outline of vessels of all types is often required. With paraffin-embedded tissues Weigert's long elastin stain shows clear definition of the elastin of vessel walls and allows the assessment of collagen accumulation. With plastic, this technique produces messy staining and Gomori's aldehyde fuchsin stain for elastin is preferable; this also works well with paraffin-embedded tissues.

## X. STAINS FOR AMYLOID

The standard stains for amyloid, namely Thioflavine T, Crystal Violet, and Congo Red, all will be positive in the majority of cases of renal amyloidosis. The occasion of amyloid in the kidney is more accurate if a combination of these stains is performed on different sections and the Congo Red preparation should be viewed in a polarizing microscope. Alternatively, EM will determine the presence or absence of amyloid. Ultrastructural examination of renal tissue remains the definitive method for the diagnosis of amyloidosis.

## XI. ADDITIONAL STAINS

Some biopsies require the application of additional stains in common use, e.g., Perl's reaction for hemosiderin or Von Kossa's stain for calcium. These techniques are available in the standard text books on histopathological techniques.

## XII. EM

Our experience has paralleled that of Siegel et al.[11] as regards the routine electron microscopic examination of renal biopsies. They showed that EM indicated a substantially different diagnosis in 11% of biopsies examined. In approximately ⅓ of the cases examined by Siegel et al. ultrastructural studies provided important information by substantiating the light microscopy diagnosis. Additional information establishing a clinically relevant classification and documenting changes occurring during the natural course of the disease was also gained.

Examples of renal diseases where electron microscope examination is mandatory are minimal change lesion (lipoid nephrosis), Alport's syndrome, occult renal involvement by systemic lupus erythaematosus, and benign familial essential hematuria.[12] However, it is beyond the scope of this monograph to provide a detailed account of the ultrastructural changes in renal disease which are available elsewhere.[8,13-16]

EM can further establish or confirm the diagnosis suggested by light microscopy especially where no renal tissue has been submitted for immunofluorescence.[12] Early membranous glomerulonephritis, mesangial IgA disease, and the dense deposit variety of membrano-proliferative glomerulonephritis amongst other conditions are instances where ultrastructural examination can be very rewarding.

As with light microscopy, the silver methenamine staining method defines basement membrane ultrastructure with sharper clarity than the standard lead and uranium stains. We have applied this technique in the ultrastructural examination of our biopsy material for several years. It has been particularly helpful in delineating subtle basement membrane changes such as early "fraying" as occurs in focal segmental sclerosis and/or hyalinosis. On several occasions, it has demonstrated early epimembranous "spike" formation in membranous glomerulonephritis that might otherwise have been overlooked.

## REFERENCES


1. **Pollack, A. D.,** Some observations on the pathology of systemic Lupus Erythaematosus, *J. Mt. Sinai Hosp. N. Y.*, 26, 224, 1959.
2. **McManus, J. F.,** The periodic acid routine applied to the kidney, *Am. J. Pathol.*, 24, 643, 1948.
3. International committee for nomenclature and noscology of renal disease, *A Handbook of Kidney Nomenclature and Noscology*, Little, Brown, Boston, 1975, 62.
4. **Heptinstall, R. H.,** *Pathology of the Kidney*, Vol. 2, 2nd ed., Little, Brown, Boston, 1974, 766.
5. **Cotran, R. S.,** Interstitial nephritis, in *Kidney Disease: Present Status*, I.A.P. Monogr. 20, Churg, J., Spargo, B.H., Mostofi, F. K., and Abell, M.R., Eds., Williams and Wilkins, Baltimore, 1979, 271.
6. **Cohen, A. H.,** Masson's trichrome stain in the evaluation of renal biopsies, *Am. J. Clin, Pathol.*, 65, 631, 1976.
7. **Jones, D. E.,** Nephrotic glomerulonephritis, *Am. J. Pathol.*, 33, 313, 1957.
8. **Burkholder, P. M.,** *Atlas of Human Glomerular Pathology*, Harper and Row, Hagerstown, Md., 1974, chap. 1.
9. **Ehrenrich, T., and Espinosa, T.,** Chromotrope silver methenamine stain of glomerular lesions, *Am. J. Clin. Pathol.*, 56, 448, 1971.
10. **Lendrum, A. G., Fraser, D. S., Slidder, W., and Henderson, R.,** Studies on the character and staining of fibrin, *J. Clin. Pathol.*, 15, 401, 1962.
11. **Siegel, N. J., Spargo, B. H., Kashgarian, M., and Hayslett, J. P.,** An evaluation of routine electron microscopy in the examination of renal biopsies, *Nephron*, 10, 209, 1973.
12. **Ryan, G. B.,** Electron microscopy in diagnostic and experimental renal pathology, *Pathology*, 10 (Abstr.), 186, 1978.
13. **Churg, J. and Grishman, E.,** Electronmicroscopy of glomerulonephritis in *Glomerulonephritis, Current Topics in Pathology* Vol. 61, Gundmann, E., Ed., Springer-Verlag, Berlin, 1976, 107.
14. **Kincaid-Smith, P.,** in *The Kidney, a Clinicopathological Study*, Blackwell, Oxford, 1975.
15. **Spargo, B. H. and Seymour, A. E.,** The value of electorn microscopy in the study of glomerular disease in *Renal Disease*, 4th ed., Black, D.A.K. and Jones, N.F., Eds., Blackwell, Oxford, 1979, chap. 8.
16. **Zollinger, H. U. and Mihatsch, M. J.,** *Renal Pathology in Biopsy*, Springer-Verlag, Berlin, 1978.

Chapter 6

# IMMUNOFLUORESCENCE AND IMMUNOPEROXIDASE PROCEDURES

**David E. Allen and John P. Dowling**

## TABLE OF CONTENTS



## I. INTRODUCTION

Labeled antibody procedures have an important place in the interpretation of the renal biopsy. These methods utilize the specific reaction of an antibody with its antigen for the localization of tissue antigens which may have diagnostic significance. In order to render the antibody-antigen combination visible, the externally added component (usually the antibody in renal histopathology) is labeled either with a fluorescent dye or with an enzyme. In the former case the labeled combination is directly visible in a fluorescence microscope while the latter method requires a subsequent histochemical reaction to render the reaction site visible. Some excellent reviews of this topic have been published[1-3] and a variety of both types of labels are available. We shall confine our discussion to the most commonly used labels, fluorescein and horseradish peroxidase (HRP).

The immunofluorescent and immunoperoxidase methods are complimentary in that both are designed to yield the same information from the biopsy. A number of studies have demonstrated the applicability of both methods to renal biopsy studies and have suggested good correlation between the methods.[1-6] The choice of whether one or other (or both) of the techniques is used therefore depends on other factors.

The choice may be made on consideration of the type of tissue section that is available. Immunoperoxidase procedures may be carried out on both frozen and paraffin sections, but in general, immunofluorescent methods are restricted to fresh-frozen sctions. Procedures for carrying out fluorescent methods on fixed or even paraffin embedded tissues have been described,[6-9] but they tend to be capricious and cannot yet be recommended for biopsy work.

Providing a good cryostat and freezing equipment (Chapter 1) are available, frozen section methods have the important advantages of simplicity and speed. Fluorescent methods can make full use of this simplicity and a biopsy can be screened for a range of antigens in several hours. However, the preparations are impermanent and demand the use of a fluorescence microscope. Also, the morphology of frozen sections is frequently poor and this can make the localization of immune deposits difficult.

Immunoperoxidase methods can be made extrememly sensitive and they yield permanent preparations which can be viewed in an ordinary microscope. In our opinion, these advantages are best utilized through the use of paraffin sections. When applied to frozen sections, immunoperoxidase methods are more time consuming than equivalent fluorescent procedures and often show increased nonspecific background staining. Also, full use cannot be made of the high resolution of peroxidase procedures because of the often poor morphology of the sections. In contrast, paraffin sections permit all of these advantages to be realized. Familiar counterstains can also be applied to enhance morphological features and the excellent storage characteristics of paraffin blocks allows retrospective studies to be made.

At the present time, immunomethods cannot routinely be applied to tissue embedded in plastic as some antigenic sites are modified or destroyed by the embedding process. It is possible that this difficulty may be overcome, at least for glycol methacrylate embedments, in the future.[10,11]

We have chosen to use commercially raised and labeled antisera for our biopsy studies. There is no doubt that better results in terms of reduced nonspecific staining and increased clarity of specific staining can be obtained through the use of custom raised and purified antisera. However, considerable time, expertise and facilities are required and these are not available to most diagnostic laboratories. Poorly prepared antisera will of course produce results inferior to the commercial products. Very good results can be obtained with commercial sera from reliable sources (e.g., DAKO, Calbiochem-Hoechst) providing careful attention is paid to experimental procedure and the use of controls (see below).

A variety of experimental procedures is available for both immunofluorescent and immunoperoxidase studies. The simplest or most direct procedure involves treatment of the biopsy section with a specific antiserum which is itself labeled with fluorescein or HRP. Indirect methods use a unlabeled specific antiserum, the binding of which is subsequently located with a labeled anti-immunoglobulin serum directed against the species in which the specific antiserum was raised (see Figure 1). The indirect method is more complex, but has the advantages of increased sensitivity and economy since any number of different specific antisera can be located with the one labeled anti-immunoglobulin. A third important method, the unlabeled antibody method or peroxidase antiperoxidase (PAP) method, can be used for immunoperoxidase studies. In this, an anti-immunoglobulin serum is used to combine with bound specific antiserum, as in the indirect method, but here this is not labeled. Instead it is further reacted with a peroxidase-antiperoxidase complex. This complex is a combination of HRP with an antibody to HRP produced in the same species as the specific antisera. It will thus also react with the anti-immunoglobulin serum (see Figure 1). This PAP procedure thus requires no labeled sera and is extremely sensitive. In some cases this sensitivity may exceed that of radioimmunoassay methods.

Our routine procedure for examining renal biopsies uses the direct immunofluorescent method on fresh-frozen sections. We have found this to be the most convenient and least time consuming procedure. The short processing sequence involved minimizes the risk of loss of the more labile tissue antigens (e.g., complement fractions) and the technique reliably yields results of adequate quality (Plate 4).* In cases of particular interest or difficulty, additional immunoperoxidase studies may be carried out using the PAP procedure (Plate 5).* This is done on the portion of the biopsy reserved for optical microscopy if this was processed into paraffin. Alternatively, residual tissue from the frozen block is carefully fixed and processed into paraffin. Full details of these procedures are

* Plates 4 and 5 appear following page 88.

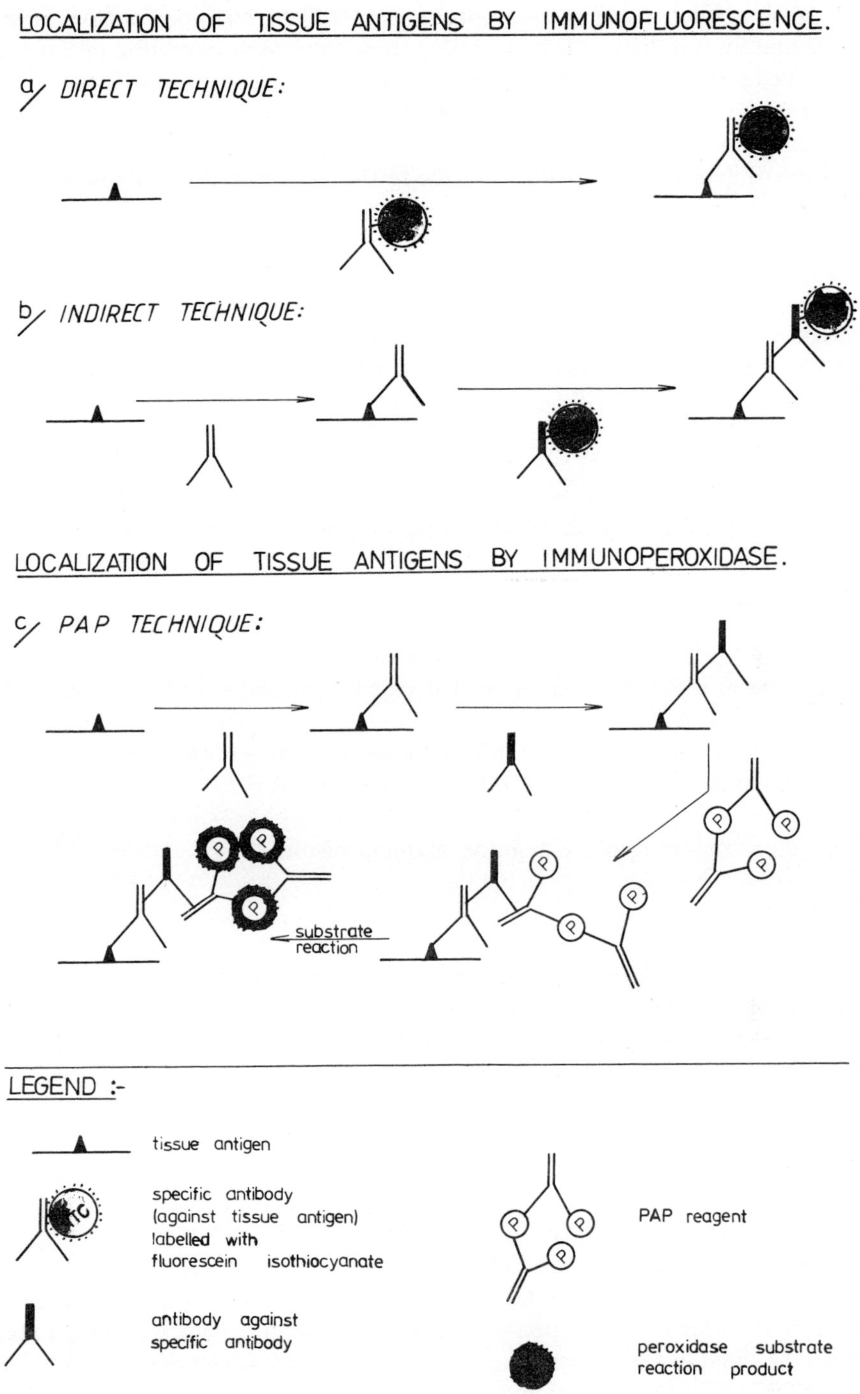


FIGURE 1. Diagramatic representation of immunohistochemical reactions.

set out below. In addition, an example of an indirect immunofluorescent procedure is given. This may occasionally be useful when a particular labeled antiserum is unavailable.

In order to derive maximum information and benefit from fluorescent preparations, it is important that they be examined with properly selected equipment which is correctly operated. Many, if not most, hospital laboratories will be equipped with a fluorescent microscope and be familiar with its use. For those who require additional information or who may be beginners in the field an excellent practical account of suitable equipment and its operation is given by Nairn.[12] Information on particular equipment is also available from the manufacturer.

The review by Nairn also provides a guide to the photography of immunofluorescent preparations. Although similar in most respects to standard brightfield photomicrography, fluorescent preparations usually demand the use of fast film if overlong exposure times are to be avoided. We have found high-speed Ektachrome® film (Kodak®) to be most suitable for this purpose and routinely use Ektachrome® 200 (Daylight). This material has a rated speed of 200 ASA, but may be specially processed to give a speed of 600 ASA. Full details of processing are available from the manufacturers.

## II. IMMUNOFLUORESCENT TECHNIQUES

### A. Control Preparations[13]

Immunohistological specificity of the conjugated reagents may be determined by the use of several controls:

1. Incubation of the tissue section with fluorescein isothiocyanate (FITC)-labeled antibody adsorbed with the specific antigen
2. Incubation of the tissue with unlabeled specific antibodies to block specifically the antigenic sites before addition of the fluorescent antibodies
3. Incubation of the tissue with FITC-labeled normal gamma globulin or gamma globulin containing antibodies to an unrelated antigen

All these steps should produce negative staining results.

### B. Direct Method

1. The snap-frozen biopsy portion is removed from cold storage and, using chilled instruments, rapidly transferred to the prechilled microtome chuck which is layered with a polyethylene glycol counting medium (e.g., OCT compound, Tissue-Tek). The tissue must not be allowed to thaw. This assembly is rapidly quenched in liquid nitrogen (or $CO_2$/ethanol) to complete attachment of the tissue to the chuck.
2. The chuck is placed on the cryostat microtome and the block allowed to equilibrate to $-18/-25°C$. Sections are then cut at 6$\mu$m using the antiroll plate to ensure flatness. The sections are transferred to separate slides at room temperature and allowed to dry either at room temperature for 30 min or in a current of air at 0 to 4°C for 2 hr. The number of sections required will depend on the range of antigens being screened (see Chapter 7). Fixation is not required. It is advisable to mark the area of the section on the back of the slide with a diamond marker.
3. Place the slides in a chamber which can be kept moist. Cover the area of the section with FITC (fluorescein isothiocyanate) labeled antihuman serum diluted with phosphate buffered saline (PBS)*. A perspex tray containing strips of plastic foam to support the slides and fitted with a lid is readily made. The foam is kept damp with water to provide humidity. The optimum dilution of the sera will vary from batch to batch. Usually the manufacturer will give a recommended figure and this

* PBS consists of: 8.5 g sodium chloride, 1.07 g disodium hydrogen phosphate (anhyd), 2nd 0.39 g sodium dihydrogen phosphate ($2H_20$). Distilled water to 1 ℓ.

is a useful starting point. If background staining is troublesome, increase the dilution of the sera. If known positive control sections are available, the optimum dilution of the sera may be determined as the highest dilution giving well defined positive results. The sera may be applied using a fine Pasteur pipette or a wire loop. It is possible to store diluted antisera for serveral weeks at 4°C. Sections of the biopsy used as controls are treated with a nonimmune conjugate (−ve, control) or with immune conjugated serum against an ubiquitous plasma protein such as albumin (+ve, control).

4. Leave the slides in a moist atmosphere for 20 min at room temperature. Rinse, drain, and wash with 2 × 5 min changes of PBS and mount in buffered glycerol (pH 8.6).
5. It is advantageous if the staining tray can be gently agitated on a mechanical shaker during the washing process. Examine the slides by UV and narrow band blue fluorescence microscopy.

### C. Indirect Method

1. Prepare frozen sections as in the above method.
2. Layer over the sections the diluted unlabeled specific antiserum. Leave for 20 min and wash as above.
3. Drain and carefully remove excess PBS with tissue or filter paper, and layer on FITC labeled anti-IgG to the species in which the primary serum was raised. Leave for 20 min and wash as above.
4. Mount the slides in buffered glycerol (pH 8.6) and examine in the fluorescence microscope.

## III. PAP — IMMUNOPEROXIDASE TECHNIQUE

It is recommended that this method be applied to paraffin sections prepared according to the processing sequence detailed in Chapter 3. If desired, fresh frozen tissue originally prepared for immunofluorescence may be transferred to Duboscq-Brasil fixtive (without thawing) and subsequently processed into paraffin.

Prepare 2 to 4 μm paraffin sections as described in Chapter 3. Bring the sections to water and incubate sequentially in the following solutions:

| | | |
|---|---|---|
| 1. | 0.2% hydrochloric acid (HCl) in methanol (destroys endogenous peroxidase activity) | 30 min |
| 2. | Rinse in distilled water | |
| 3. | Equilibrate in 0.05 *M* Tris-HCl buffer (pH 7.6) | 15 min |
| 4. | Apply 1:10 normal swine serum to block nonspecific binding, use the apparatus described above for direct immunofluorescence; dilute the serum with PBS | 10 min |
| 5. | Wash in 0.1 *M* glycine-NaOH buffer (pH 9.5) | 15 min |
| 6. | Equilibrate with 0.05 *M* Tris-HCl buffer (pH 7.6); Steps 5 and 6 are preferably carried out on a mechanically shaken table | 10 min |
| 7. | Apply specific rabbit antiserum to human component diluted 1:20 with PBS | 60 min |
| 8. | Wash as in Steps 5 and 6 above | |
| 9. | Apply swine antirabbit IgG diluted 1:40 | 60 min |
| 10. | Wash as in Steps 5 and 6 above | |
| 11. | Apply rabbit PAP complex diluted 1:40 | 60 min |
| 12. | Wash as in Steps 5 and 6 above | |
| 13. | Develop the peroxidase activity by treating with 0.05% diaminobenzidine tetrahydrochloride* in 0.05 *M* Tris-HCl buffer (pH 7.6) and containing 0.01% hydrogen peroxidase; carry out this step in the dark | 30 min |

* Caution: diaminobenzidine may be a carcinogen.

14. Wash in 0.05 *M* Tris-HCl buffer (pH 7.6) 5 min
15. Counterstain as desired
16. Dehydrate, clear, and mount

The dilutions given above are provided as a starting point. They can be exceeded with advantage if high quality sera are available.

The above procedure contains a number of steps designed to minimize background staining. These are the destruction of endogenous peroxidase activity, preliminary treatment with nonimmune sera, and washing with a high pH buffer. Other methods to enhance the sensitivity of the PAP procedure have been described. These include pronase pretreatment of sections,[14] trypsin pretreatment,[7,15] and the use of special fixative solutions.[16] We have not tested these methods with renal biopsies.

## REFERENCES

1. **Taylor, C. R.,** Immunoperoxidase techniques, *Arch. Pathol. Lab. Med.,* 102, 113, 1978.
2. **Petts, V. and Roitt, I. M.,** Peroxidase conjugates for the demonstration of tissue antibodies: evaluation of the technique, *Clin. Exp. Immunol.,* 9, 407, 1971.
3. **Burns, J.,** Immunohistological methods and their application in the routine laboratory, in *Recent Advances in Histopathology.,* No. 10, Anthony, P. P. and Woolf, N., Eds., Churchill Livingstone, Edinburgh, 1978, chap. 16.
4. **Davey, M. D. and Busch, G. J.,** Immunohistochemistry of glomerulonephritis using horseradish peroxidase and fluorescein labelled antibody, *Am. J. Pathol.,* 53, 531, 1970.
5. **Elias, J. M. and Miller, F.,** A comparison of the unlabeled enzyme method with immunofluorescence for the evaluation of human immunologic renal disease, *Am. J. Clin. Pathol.,* 64, 464, 1975.
6. **Denk, H., Syré, G., and Weirich, E.,** Immunomorphologic methods in routine pathology. Application of immunofluorescence and the unlabeled antibody-enzyme (peroxidase-antiperoxidase) technique to formalin fixed, paraffin embedded kidney biopsies, *Beitr. Pathol.,* 160, 187, 1977.
7. **Curran, R. C. and Gregory, J.,** The unmasking of antigens in paraffin sections of tissue by trypsin, *Experientia,* 15, 1300, 1977.
8. **Burns, R. B. and Anderson, A. C.,** Dioxan in paraffin embedding for immunofluorescence, *Med. Lab. Sci.,* 35, 99, 1978.
9. **Dorsett, B. H. and Ioachim, H. L.,** A method for the use of immunofluorescence on paraffin embedded tissue, *Am. J. Clin. Pathol.,* 69, 66, 1978.
10. **Craig Spaur, R. and Moriarty, G. C.,** Improvements of Glycol Methacrylate, *J. Histochem. Cytochem.,* 25, 163, 1977.
11. **Scotto, J.,** Immunofluorescence on resin-embedded material, *Histopathology,* 1, 371, 1977.
12. **Nairn, R. C.,** *Fluorescent Protein Tracing,* Churchill Livingstone, London, 1976.
13. **Spiegelberg, H. L.,** Principles of methods in *Textbook of Immunopathology,* Vol. 2, 2nd ed., Miescher, P. A. and Muller-Eberhard, H. J., Eds., Grune & Stratton, New York, 1976, 1114.
14. **Denk, H., Radaszkiewicz, T., and Weirich, E.,** Pronase pretreatment of tissue sections enhances sensitivity of the unlabeled antibody-enzyme (PAP) technique *J. Immunol. Methods,* 15, 163, 1977.
15. **Hautzer, N. W., Wittkuhn, J. F., and Elliott McCoughey, W. T.,** Trypsin digestion in immunoperoxidase staining, *J. Histochem. Cytochem.,* 28, 52, 1980.
16. **McLean, I. W. and Nakane, P. K.,** Periodate-lysine-paraformaldehyde fixative. A new fixative for immunoelectron microscopy, *J. Histochem. Cytochem.,* 22, 1077, 1974.

Chapter 7

# CLINICAL RELEVANCE OF IMMUNOHISTOCHEMICAL TECHNIQUES

**David E. Allen and John P. Dowling**

The simplicity of direct immunofluorescence performed with reagents of high quality makes this the method of choice in most laboratories dealing with renal biopsies. Other workers prefer the technique of indirect immunofluorescence with its increased sensitivity. The most sensitive results with immunoperoxidase labeling are achieved using frozen unfixed renal tissue, but nonspecific background staining causes considerable problems with both the fresh-frozen and fixed material; this remains a difficult problem to overcome (see Chapter 6).

Immunoperoxidase techniques have proved particularly useful when the tissue selected for immunofluorescence has been inadequate or insufficient. The nature of the fixative used for light microscopy has an important bearing on the application of this method. But, in general, formalin- or Duboscq-Brasil-fixed tissues, even after processing into paraffin, retain sufficient reactivity to provide results.

Immunohistochemical techniques provide the pathologist with a means of further classifying and assessing renal disease. The immunopathogenesis of many of the glomerulonephritidies is now well established.[1] In general terms two basic patterns of immunoglobulin deposition are detected in most cases of glomerulonephritis. One, accounting for approximately 4 to 5% of adult cases of glomerulonephritis, is the linear deposition of IgG usually associated with a crescentic nephritis. This pattern indicates the presence of antiglomerular basement membrane antibodies present both in the glomeruli and in the serum. The latter may be detected by radioimmunoassay or the much less precise technique of indirect immunofluorescence using normal fresh-frozen renal tissue and the patient's serum.[2,3] Recently, the linear deposition of IgA has been described in a patient with crescentic nephritis associated with lung hemorrhage (Goodpasture's syndrome.)[4] This condition had previously been linked with the IgG antiglomerular basement membrane antibodies only. Other conditions with a linear IgG pattern outlining glomerular basement membrane are lupus nephritis, diabetes mellitus, hypothyroidism, renal transplants, and in some cases of lipoid nephrosis associated with heroin addiction; in most instances these examples provide light linear staining only (see Table 1).

The second pattern evident in approximately 80% of an adult nephritic population is one of granular deposition of immunoglobulins and complement in particular.[5] When such deposits are seen distributed over the peripheral aspect of the glomerular capillary loops they are considered to denote an immune complex-based glomerulonephritis. While circulating soluable immune complexes composed of antigen and specific antibody are deposited in the glomerulus to initiate and often prolong the development of many types of glomerulonephritis, recent experimental work suggest that in some forms of nephritis immune complexes are formed *in situ* within the glomerulus itself. It is postulated that fixed or "planted" foreign tissue antigens combine with circulating specific antibodies to form the complexes responsible for the glomerular reaction. Such a mechanism may be implicated in poststreptococcal glomerulonephritis.[6]

The deposition of complement components in a wide variety of glomerular diseases and the experimental modulation of glomerular reactions by such methods as cobra venom factor impairment of complement activity indicate a central role for this complex series of serum proteins.[7] The activation of this system proceeds via two mechanisms,

**Table 1**
**DIFFERENTIAL DIAGNOSIS OF IMMUNOHISTOCHEMICAL PATTERNS**

| Pattern | Disease morphology | Proteins deposited | Differentiating features |
|---|---|---|---|
| Diffuse granular outlining glomerular capillary loops | Membranous GN[a] Ideopathic Secondary | IgG > IgM > IgA; $C_3$; also fibrin; early stages: regular fine-coarse; later: maybe uneven, less intense; fibrin: usually eight deposits | Ideopathic and secondary types show similar pattern; membranous pattern has preceded development of anti-GBM[b] GN[16] are followed diffuse proliferative GN[17] |
| | Edocapillary (post-infectious) GN | IgG > IgM > IgA; fine-coarse; irregular distribution $C_3$ usually with IgG $C_3$ maybe only deposit; fibrin maybe present | Pattern produced by wide variety of different antigens;[1] mesangial staining also seen to varying degree; fibrin may present in capillary loops and increscents if present |
| | Diffuse proliferative lupus GN | IgG+/−IgM+/−IgA; $C_3$ and Clq—(usually); fibrin usually seen in capillary loops | Mesangial staining usually seen; irregular tubular basement membranes and peritubular vessels may show Ig[c] and C[d] deposits. |
| | Mesangiocapillary GN a. Subendothelial deposit type (1) | IgG > IgM > IgA; $C_3$: irregular distribution, fine and coarse deposits; Clq may be present | Mesangial (especially with $C_3$) staining often prominent with lobular appearance; froperdin also deposited |
| | b. Dense deposit type (2) | Mainly $C_3$: heavy "ribbon-like" outline of GMB; Clq in small amounts; scattered IgG, IgM, and IgA | Distinctive large granular mesangial deposits of $C_3$ usually seen; Ig staining is sparse; thrioflavine T stain is positive[18] |
| | c. "Secondary" type (1) with extensive GBM "splitting" | Variety of patterns of Ig granular deposits; $C_3$ usually heavy | The "secondary" causes include: systemic lupus erythaematosus, Henoch-Schönlein purpura; polyarteritis nodosa, polyarthritis, polymositis, some cryoglobulinaemias, hepatitis Bvirus, drug addicts, ventriculo-atrial shunts, $C_2$ deficiency; chronic candida speticemia, malaria, toxic epidermal necrolysis (Lyell), sickle cell anaemia, post-streptococcal GN, partial lipo-dystrophy (usually dense deposit variety) |

| | | | |
|---|---|---|---|
| Diffuse granular mainly mesangial | "Mesangial IgA nephropathy"<br>a. Minor glomerular lesions<br>b. Focal segmental proliferative GN<br>c. Diffuse mesnagial proliferative GN<br>d. Focal segmental sclerosis +/− hyalinosis. (+/− mesangial proliferation) | IgA: predominantly in mesangium but some irregular staining of peripheral capillary loops may be seen; +/− IgG, IgM; $C_3$: as for IgA; Clq: suggests lupus GN | Fibrin, previously considered an indicator of Henoch-Schönlein purpura, is seen in IgA nephrophaty", suggesting that these entities are part of one disease spectrum";[19] Clq is negative in "mesangial IgA nephropathy; cirrhosis and some examples of acute liver disease are associated with GN, mostly mesangial proliferative; mesangial IgA and $C_3$ are charactistically found in them; IgA is found in cutaneous capillaries in many cases of "mesangial IgA nephrophathy", Henoch-Schönlein purpura,[20] and alcoholic liver disease[21] |
| | Diffuse mesangial proliferative GN | IgM and $C_3$—moderately heavy deposits | Pattern associated with nephrotic syndrome[12] |
| | Mild lupus nephritis—focal or diffuse | IgG and $C_3$—mainly mesangial staining | |
| Diffuse linear GBM +/− TBM[e] staining | Diffuse crescentic GN (+/− pulmonary hemorrhage); focal segmental proliferative and necrotizing GN;[23] diffuse mesangial proliferative GN | IgG normally heavily evenly outlining GBM; (+/− TBM); rarely IgA;[4] $C_3$ may show areas of linear GBM staining; $C_3$ and IgM are deposited with a fine granular pattern in some cases | TBM staining is seen in some biopsies only; similar, but usually less intense, IgG linear GBM (+/− TBM) staining may be seen in: diabetes mellitus, hypothyroidism, lupus nephritis, renal transplants, some examples of heroin nephropathy with minimal change lesion,[22] as an artefact |
| Diffuse crescentic staining with fibrin | Diffuse crescentric GN (RPGN) | Fibrin outlining glomerular crescents. | Fibrin more likely to be seen with active cellular crescents |
| | a. Anti-GBM | IgG linear outlining of GBM | |
| | b. Immune complex | IgG, IgM, IgA, $C_3$ in varying combination outlined | |
| | c. No Ig or C | Only fibrin in crescents | A variable percentage of cases of diffuse crescentic GN is negative for Ig and C[24] |
| Focal segmental granular staining | Focal and segmental proliferative GN<br>a. Ideopathic<br>b. Associated with systemic diseases | IgG, IgM, IgA, $C_3$ within mesangium and/or periphery of capillary loops; ± fibrin in crescents and involved capiallary loops | In the ideopathic variety IgM may be more evident than IgG; IgA is infrequently present; fibrin is frequently the only protein deposited in the microscopic form of polyarteritis nodosa; focal lupus nephritis can show a wide variety of patterns[25] |

**Table 1 (continued)**
**DIFFERENTIAL DIAGNOSIS OF IMMUNOHISTOCHEMICAL PATTERNS**

| Pattern | Disease morphology | Proteins deposited | Differentiating features |
|---|---|---|---|
| Focal segmental granular staining (continued) | Focal and segmental hyalinosis ±/− sclerosis | IgM and $C_3$ in segment lesions large deposits; Clq sometimes seen | Nonsclerotic glomeruli show either no deposits on IgM; $C_3$ in small amounts in the mesagnium; similar focal, semental deposits of IgM and $C_3$ may be superimposed on other patterns, e.g., membranous GN, "mesangial IgA nephropathy" as a secondary phenomenon |
| Focal/diffuse tubular basement membrane staining | Interstitial nephritis with eosinophils and/or mononuclear inflammatory cell interstitial infiltration | Variable linear/granular staining of IgG and $C_3$ | Rare examples of antibiotic-related interstitial nephritis show linear staining;[6] most are negative; Antibodies to TBM found in renal allografts and occasional patients with immune complex GN[6] |
| | Wide variety of different renal disease, e.g., various glomerulonephritides, transplants, chronic atrophic pyelonophritis | $C_3$ granular deposits | Very commonly seen, but are nonspecific |
| Focal diffuse nonspecific staining | Many "non-glomerular" diseases; "normal" kidneys; minimal change lesion (lipoid nephrosis) | IgM, $C_3$: Small granular deposits in mesangium +/− capillary loops | Very common pattern in "minor glomerular lesions" and is seen, e.g., in immediate transplant biopsies; lipoid nephrosis: deposits tend concentrate at vascular pole[24] |
| Focal/diffuse glomerular staining with fibrin predominantly | Disseminated intravascular coagulation; thrombotic thrombocytopaenic purpura; toxemic nephropathy; hemolytic uremic syndrome | Fibrin (related antigens) seen in subendothelial and mesangial regions, and as intraluminal large capillary loop microthrombi; IgM, IgG, and $C_3$: small but inconstant glomerular deposits may be seen in all these conditions[1] | Fibrin may be seen in a wide range of glomerular diseases, but it is usually the predominant protein(s) deposited in the coagulopathies; arteriolar/arterial staining may be seen; the presence/absence of fibrin probably depends on the timing of the renal biopsy[26] |

| | | | |
|---|---|---|---|
| Vascular staining | Arteritits/arteriolitis | IgG, +/− IgM, +/− IgA, $C_3$,Clq in vessel walls | Glomerular staining with Ig, C, and fibrin may accompany these vascular deposits |
| | Scleroderma | IgM IgG; $C_3$, Clq, and fibrin | Scleroderma: variable inconsistent staining of vessels; glomerular deposits of Ig and C may be seen[25] |
| | Vascular hyaloinosis | $C_3$ especially IgM and Clq also seen | Very frequent finding in many different renal diseases |

[a] Glomerulonephritis.
[b] Glomerular basement membrane.
[c] Immunoglobulin.
[d] Complement.
[e] Tubular basement membrane.

namely, the "classical" pathway initiated by immune complexes and other substances utilizing the early complement components $C_1$, $C_4$, and $C_2$; the "alternative" pathway involving the properdin system is activated by such substances as aggregated IgA, endotoxin, lipopolysaccharide, and nephritic factor acting on $C_3$, by-passing $C_1$, $C_4$, and $C_2$.

The accumulation of $C_3$ and related proteins results in the formation of the later elements of the "complement cascade", $\overline{C_3\ C_5\ C_6}$ with anaphylactoid, leucotactic, immunoadherent and opsonizing activities and $\overline{C_7\ C_8\ C_9}$, a complex producing cell lysis. These latter reactions form part of the glomerular response to injury. The recent demonstration of $C_3$ receptors on glomerular podocytes raises interesting but as yet unanswered questions regarding immune injury in glomerulonephritis.[8] It is possible that these receptors help localize complement-fixing immunocomplexes to the subepithelial region in conditions such as membranous or lupus glomerulonephritis.[9]

It has become almost standard practice to include the following panel of specific antisera, either with FITC-or peroxidase-labeles, to examine renal tissue:

**IgA** — Glomerular deposition of this immunoglobulin, secreted mostly from mucosal surfaces, is seen in a wide variety of glomerulonephritidies, idiopathic, and secondary to systemic diseases. Berger and Hinglais[10] first recognized the importance of the mesangial deposition of IgA to deline an increasingly important subgroup of nephritic patients. However, this mesangial deposition is by no means specific for "IgA nephropathy" (see Table 1). In general, IgA deposits are a specific indication of a glomerulonephritic reaction. Glomerular deposition is usually granular, but recently, as indicated above, linear staining of the glomerular basement membrane has been described in Goodpasture's syndrome.[4]

**IgG** —The presence of this immunoglobulin within glomeruli too points to a glomerulonephritic process for it is rarely seen at this site in nonglomerular diseases. IgG antitubular basement membranes may occur in association with antiglomerular basement membrane antibodies or, rarely, in isolation.[11]

**IgM** — Again IgM is deposited in most forms of glomerulonephritis but is less specific. While is activates the classical pathway of complement, aggregated IgM nonspecifically binds $C_3$; both IgM and $C_3$ are frequently positive in nonglomerular diseases. Moderate to heavy mesangial IgM aggregates associated with $C_3$ have been found in some patients with a nephrotic syndrome showing mesangial proliferative glomerulonephritis.[12] Small amounts of IgM are found in some cases of minimal change lesion (lipoid nephrosis) while larger segmental deposits occuring in association with $C_3$ and Clq strongly suggest a diagnosis of focal segmental hyalinosis and/or sclerosis.

**$C_3$** — This component of complement occupies a central position in the understanding of the pathogenesis of the glomerulonephritidies. Almost all glomerulonephropathies have been demonstrated to have $C_3$ with glomeruli. The isolated deposition of $C_3$ within glomeruli is considered to indicate involvement of the alternative pathway of complement activation probably best seen in the heavy $C_3$ glomerular deposits of mesangial IgA nephropathy and membranoproliferative glomerulonephritis, (especially type II — dense deposit disease.)[13]

**Clq** — Where activation of complement precedes via the classical pathway, the early components, C1, $C_4$, and $C_2$ are utilized. The glomerular deposition of Clq is a more reliable indicator of such activation occurring in many glomerular diseases than is $C_4$. Classical pathway activation is frequently seen in such conditions as in nephritis of systemic lupus and Henoch-Schönlein purpura.

**Fibrin** — In glomerular disease, activation of coagulation factors takes place by the intrinsic mechanism involving Hageman factor via surface contact. Immune complexes or alternative pathway activators of complement further result in the formation of fibrin or fibrin-realted antigens. These proteins are frequently deposited in glomerular and nonglomerular diseases. They are seen in association with immune complexes as insudative aggregates in glomerular capillaries or larger vessels and as granular deposits in conditions such as hypertension, eclampsia, and in transplants. In disseminated intravasular coagulation large masses of fibrin-related antigens may be seen.[14]

**Albumen** — In some instances the demonstration of protein deposition in the glomeruli is the result of a nonspecific adsorptive effect. Labeled antialbumen antibodies will often be detected outlining the glomerular basement membrane in a similar manner. Anti-IgG and antialbumen are frequently seen in diabetes nephropathy with a linear pattern along with the glomerular basement membrane.

**Control** — The specificity of the conjugates will already have been determined. The use of antibody raised in animals dissimilar to those used in the test system is a further check on the nonspecific deposition of proteins.

Other conjugates employed are IgE, properdin, and $C_4$. IgE has been detected in glomeruli by some workers in the minimal change lesion (lipoid nephrosis;[15] properdin deposition indicates that complement deposition, specifically that of $C_3$, is due to the activation of the alternative pathway of complement; and $C_4$ is an indicator of the utilization of the early components of complement via the classical pathway; however, as indicated, Clq appears to be a more reliable indicator of the latter.

We have included a Table 1 outlining the major patterns of immunohistochemical staining seen in renal diseases. It also provides differential features that help distinguish the lesions demonstrated by light microscopy.

## REFERENCES


1. **Albini, B., Brentjens, J. R., and Andres, G. A.,** *The Immunopathology of the Kidney,* Current Topics in Immunology Series No. 11 in Turk, J., Ed., Arnold, London, 1979.
2. **McPhaul, J. J. and Dixon, F. J.,** The presence of Antiglomerular Antibodies in peripheral blood, *J. Immunol.,* 103, 1168, 1969.
3. **Wilson, C. B., Marquardt, H., and Dixon, F. J.,** Radioimmune Assay for circulating antiglomerular basement membrane antibodies, *Kidney Int.,* 6, 114a, 1974.
4. **Border, W. A., Baehler, R. W., Bhathena, D., and Glassock, R. J.,** IgA antibasement membrane nephritis with pulmonary haemorrhage, *Ann. Intern. Med.,* 91, 22, 1979.
5. **Dixon, F. J. and Wilson, C. B.,** Immunological renal injury produced by formation and deposition of immune complexes in *Immunologic Mechanisms of Renal Disease,* Wilson, C. B., Ed., Churchill Livingstone, New York, 1979, 10.
6. **Wilson, C. B. and Dixon, F. J.,** Renal injury from immune reactions in or of the kidney, in *Immunologic Mechanisms of Renal Disease,* Wilson, C. B., Ed., Churchill Livingstone, New York, chap. 2.
7. **Schreiber, R. D. and Müller-Eberhard, H. M.,** Complement and renal disease, in *Immunologic Mechanisms of Renal Disease,* Wilson, C. B., Ed., Churchill Livingstone, New York, chap. 3.
8. **Gelfand, M. C., Frank, M. M., and Green, I.,** A receptor for the third component of complement in the human glomerulus, *J. Exp. Med.,* 142, 1029, 1975.
9. **Shin, M. L., Gelfand, M. C., Nagle, R. B., Carlo, J. R., Green, I., and Frank, M. M.,** Localization of receptors for activated complement on visceral epithelial cells of the human glomerulus, *J. Immunol.,* 118, 869, 1977.
10. **Berger, J. and Hinglais, N.,** Les Dépôts intercapillaries d'IgA-IgG, *J. Urol. Nephrol.,* 74, 694, 1968.
11. **Wilson, C. B. and Dixon, F. J.,** Renal injury from immune reactions in or of the kidney in *Immunologic Mechanisms of Renal Disease,* Wilson, C. B., Ed., Churchill Livingstone, New York, 1979, 58.
12. **Cohen, A. H., Border, W. A., and Glassock, R. J.,** Nephrotic syndrome with glomerular mesangial IgM deposits, *Lab. Invest.,* 38, 610, 1978.

13. **West, C. D.**, Membranoproliferative glomerulonephritis (MPGN) in *Immunologically Mediated Renal Diseases — Criteria for Diagnosis and Treatment,* McCluskey, R. T. and Andres, G. A., Eds., Marcel Dekker, New York, 1978, 51.
14. **Zollinger, H. U. and Mihatsch, M. J.**, *Renal Pathology in Biopsy,* Springer-Verlag, Berlin, 1978, 164.
15. **Gerber, M. A. and Paronetto, F.**, IgE in Glomeruli of patients with nephrotic syndrome, *Lancet,* 1, 1097, 1971.
16. **Klassen, J., Elswood, L., Grossberg, A. L., Milgrom, F., Montes, M., Sepulveda, M., and Andres, G. A.**, Evolution of membranous nephropathy into Antiglomerular Basement Membrane Glomerulonephristis, *N. Engl. J. Med.,* 290, 1340, 1974.
17. **Richet, G., Fillastre, J. P., Morel-Maroger, L., and Bariety, J.**, Change from Diffuse Proliferative to Membranous Glomerulonephritis. Serial biopsies in four cases, *Kidney Int.,* 5, 57, 1974.
18. **Churg, J., Duffy, J. L., and Bernstein, J.**, Identification of dense deposit disease, *Arch. Pathol. Lab. Med.,* 103, 67, 1979.
19. **Nakamoto, Y., Assano, Y., Dohi, K., Fujioka, M., Iida, H., Kida, H., Kibe, Y., Hattori, N., and Takeuchi, J.**, Primary IgA Glomerulonephritis and Schönlein-Henoch Purpura Nephritis: clinicopathological and immunohistochemical characteristics, *Q. J. Med.,* New Series XLVII, 188, 495, 1978.
20. **Tsai, C. C., Giangiacomo, J., and Zucker, J.**, Dermal IgA Deposits in Henoch-Schönlein Purpura and Berger's Nephritis, *Lancet,* 1, 342, 1975.
21. **Kater, L., Jobbis, A. C., Baart De La Faille-Kuyper, E., Vogten, A. J., and Grijm, R.**, Alcoholic hepatic disease — specificity of IgA deposits in liver, *Am. J. Clin. Pathol.,* 71, 51, 1979.
22. **Matalon, R., Katz, L., Gall, G., Waldo, E., Cabaluna, C., and Eisinger, R. P.**, Glomerular sclerosis in adults with nephrotic syndrome, *Ann. Intern. Med.,* 80, 488, 1974.
23. **McPhaul, J. J., Jr. and Mullins, J. D.**, Glomerulonephritis mediated by antibody to glomerular basement membrane, *J. Clin. Invest.,* 57, 351, 1976.
24. **Glassock, R. J.**, Clinical features of immunologic glomerular disease, in *Immunologic Mechanisms of Renal Disease,* Wilson, C. B., Ed., Churchill Livingstone, New York, 1979, chap. 9.
25. **Jenis, E. H. and Lowenthal, D. T.**, *Kidney Biopsy Interpretation,* Davis, Philadelphia, 1977, 185.
26. **McCoy, R. C., Abramowsky, E. R., and Krueger, R.**, The hemolytic uremic syndrome and positive immunofluorescence studies, *J. Pediatr.,* 85, 170, 1974.

Chapter 8

# THE TECHNIQUE OF GLOMERULAR CULTURE

**Eric F. Glasgow, Wayne W. Hancock, and Robert C. Atkins**

## TABLE OF CONTENTS

## I. RELEVANCE OF GLOMERULAR CULTURE IN NEPHROPATHOLOGY

Glomerular culture, being such a recent investigative tool, has not yet become an integral part of renal biopsy evaluation in the same way as light microscopic, immunofluorescent, or electron microscopic techniques have become part of routine renal histopathology. Such culture has the potential to allow assessment of glomerular cells in a unique way. Already glomerular culture has revealed the macrophage as an important cell in crescentic nephritis,[7,27,39] and has provided a means of quantitating macrophages within the glomerular tuft throughout the evolution of experimental glomerulonephritis.[29,30]

As expected, the pattern of glomerular cell outgrowth in culture reflects the underlying disease process in the glomerulus in the various types of human glomerulonephritis.[7,39] Furthermore, glomerular isolation and culture will provide a method for studying the pathophysiological function of the individual glomerular cells.

The main practical problem with glomerular culture is the current lack of positive identification of the intrinsic glomerular cell types except for the macrophage. Specific glomerular cell markers will allow positive identification of the intrinsic glomerular cells which will be a big step forward both in glomerular culture and indeed in the assessment of glomerular tissue sections. We have described techniques for such glomerular marker identification although no specific antibodies are as yet available.

## II. INTRODUCTION

Tissue culture of isolated glomeruli has been developed over recent years[1-4] and is now being used as an investigative method for the study of both normal and glomerular cell function and the behavior of these cells in renal disease. The principle of glomerular culture is that freshly isolated glomeruli from many mammalian species, including man, attach to the flask surface in culture and migration of glomerular cells occurs during prolonged culture. The rate and type of glomerular outgrowth, although remarkably similar among normal animals of many species, varies with certain renal diseases in which the glomerulus is affected. Although most investigators agree that two or more different cell types are seen in the outgrowth, there is still not complete agreement on glomerular cell identification as definitive glomerular cell markers have yet to be characterized. Nevertheless, glomerular culture is becoming an important investigative tool allowing in vitro analysis of normal and diseased glomerular structure and function.

## III. SOURCES OF GLOMERULI

Kidneys from human nephrectomies and cadavers, percutaneous and surgically obtained renal biopsies,[5-8] and fetal and infant kidneys[9,10] have been used as sources of glomeruli, as well as the kidneys of many experimental animals including monkeys, sheep, rabbits, rats, and mice.[11] As in most tissue culture studies, the age of the donor tissue is important in subsequent interpretation of results, since embryonic tissues grow more rapidly and often with different characteristics than those of the adult.[10,12,13]

## IV. ISOLATION OF GLOMERULI

Isolation of glomeruli is readily achieved by a sieving technique[6,14,15] because of the marked resistance of the glomerulus to mechanical dissociation, in contrast to the remainder of the kidney. Tissues too small for easy manipulation, such as human renal

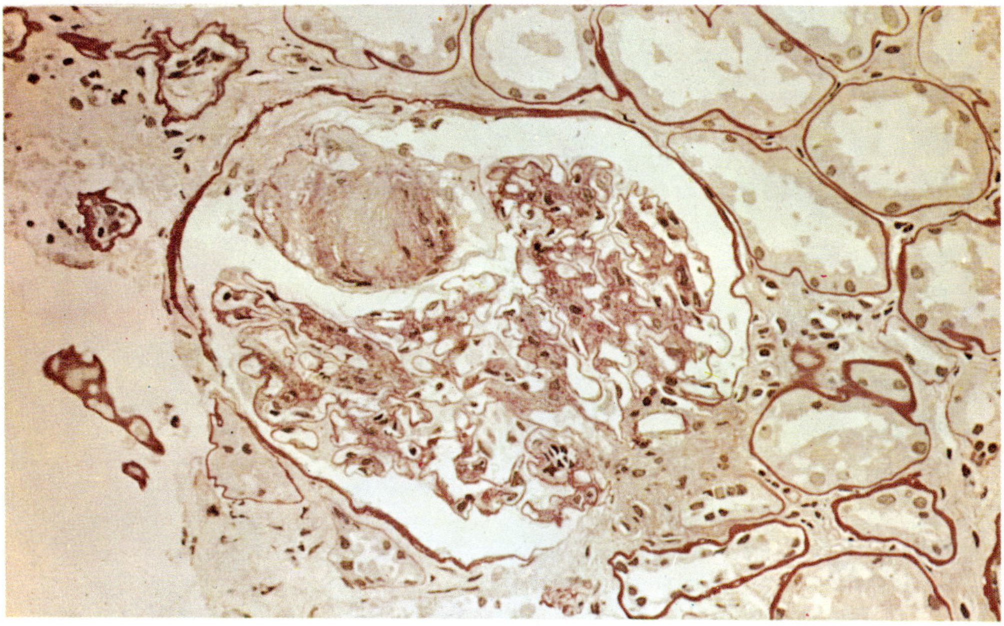

PLATE 1. Diabetic nodular (Kimmelstriel-Wilson) glomerulosclerosis. Duboscq-Brasil fixation. Spurr's resin. Periodic acid-Schiff. (Magnification × 1200, shown at 75%.)

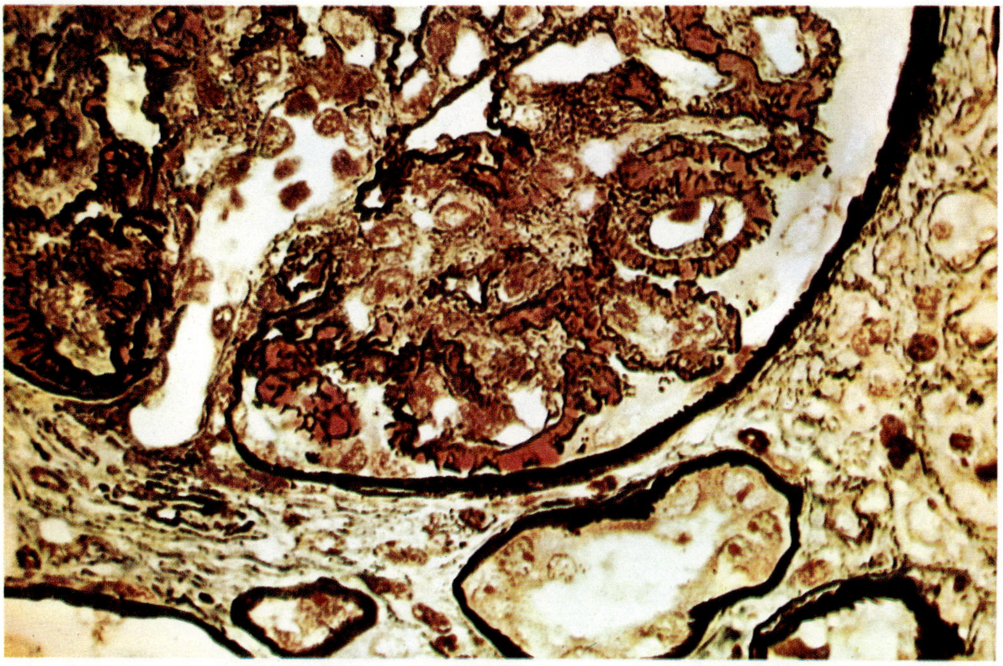

PLATE 2. Membranous glomerulonephritis showing large subepithelial protein deposits and "spike" formation with sclerotic collapse of other capillary loops. Duboscq-Brasil fixation. Spurr's resin. Silver methenamine-Masson trichrome. (Magnification, oil × 1800, shown at 75%.)

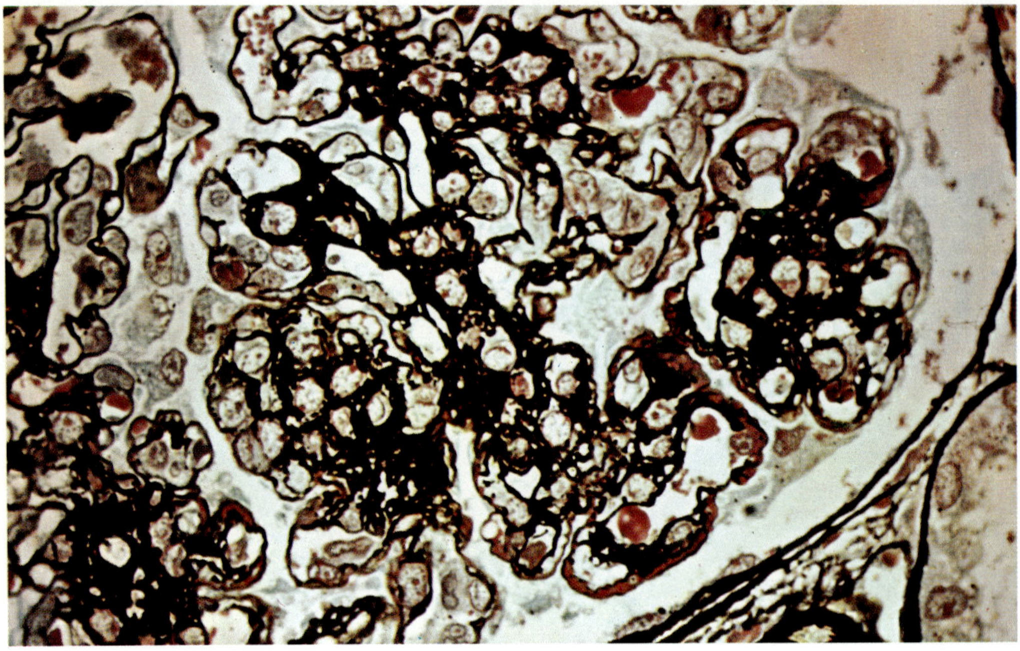

PLATE 3. Mesangiocapillary glomerulonephritis, subendothelial deposit variety (type 1) with extensive deposits, some irregular reduplication of glomerular basement membrane, and mesangial proliferation. Duboscq-Brasil fixation. Paraffin-embedded. Silver methenamine-Masson trichrome stain. (Magnification, oil ×4800, shown at 75%.)

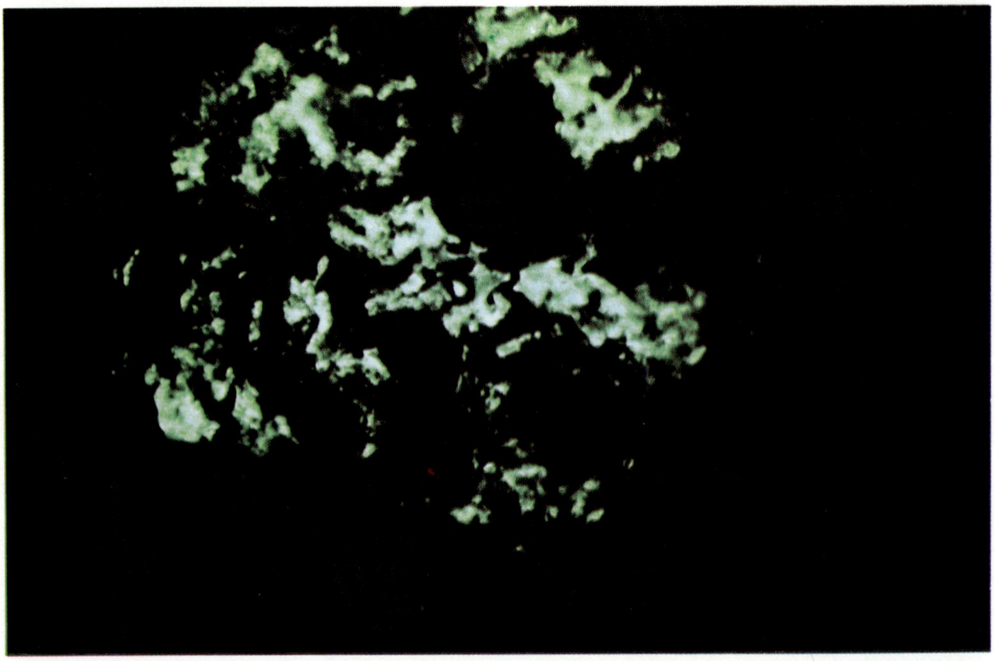

PLATE 4. Heavy IgA mesangial deposits; "IgA mesangial nephropathy". Direct immunofluorescence. (Magnification ×1800, shown at 75%.)

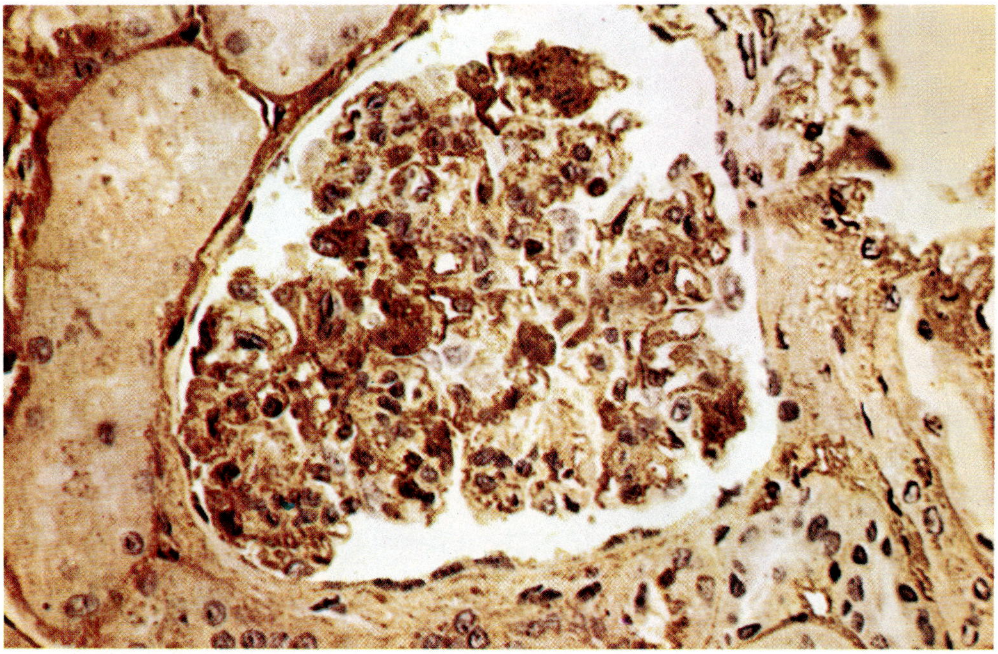

PLATE 5. Irregular deposition of IgA in mesangium and some capillary loops; biopsy from cirrhotic patient. Background interstitial and tubular basement membrane staining. P.A.P. method. Parossin section. (Magnification × 1800, shown at 75%.)

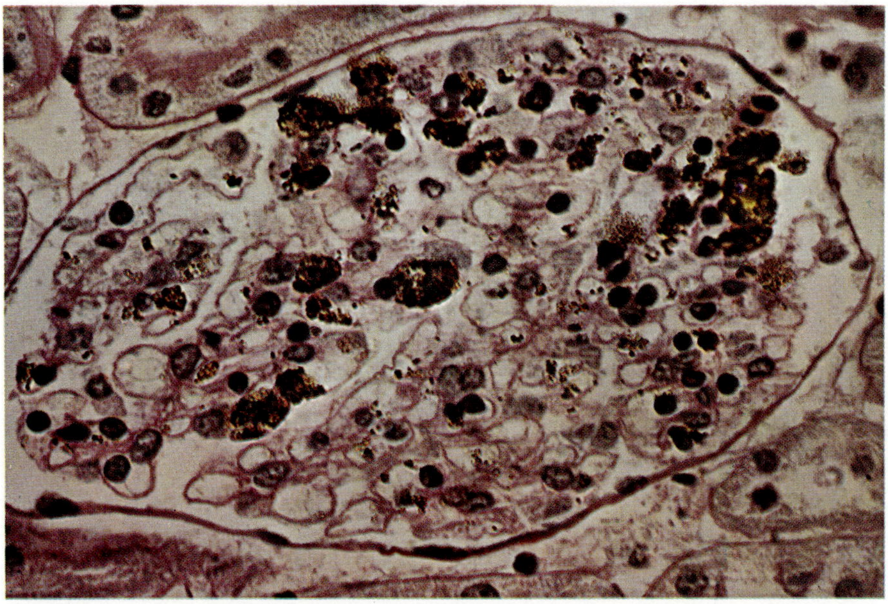

PLATE 6. PAS-stained section of rabbit renal cortex after arterial infusion of ferrous oxide demonstrates iron trapped in capillary loops. (Magnification × 1800, shown at 75%.)

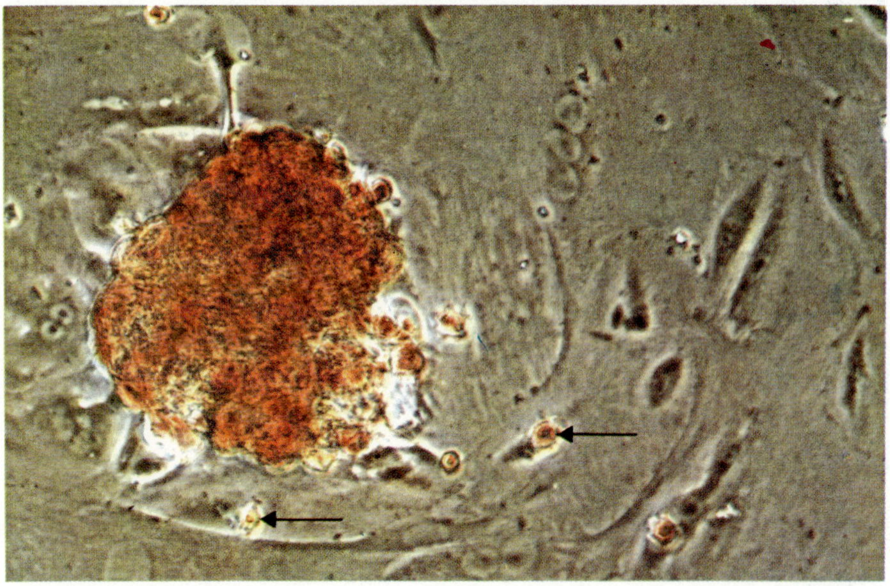

PLATE 7. Histochemical labeling by β-glucuronidase of Type III cells (arrows) seen in outgrowth from glomerulus from patient with crescentic glomerulonephritis. Labeling is also seen of monocytes within the glomerulus. (Magnification × 900, shown at 75%.)

**Table 1**
**MESH FOR RETAINING GLOMERULI OF VARIOUS SPECIES**

| Gauge | Pore size (μm) | Species |
|---|---|---|
| 60 | 250 | — |
| 80 | 184 | Sheep |
| 100 | 151 | Man, monkey |
| 120 | 128 | Dog |
| 150 | 103 | Rabbit |
| 300 | 63 | Rat, mouse |

biopsies, are isolated by microdissection. Other methods of glomerular isolation combine sedimentation or slow centrifugation with the basic sieving techniques,[2,3,16] or use of sucrose,[17] or ficoll gradients.[18]

### A. Sieving Technique

The kidneys are decapsulated using a scalpel blade, and the paler cortex removed. Cortical sections are sliced into small blocks (5-mm cubes) and placed in Medium 199 with 1% fetal calf serum (FCS) at 4°C until processing. Storage of small cubes of tissues for up to 24 hr usually results in growth in culture, but longer periods before glomerular isolation result in decreased attachment and abnormal outgrowths.[6]

The cortical cubes of tissue are processed in a laminar flow hood using sterile techniques. Cortical cubes are first minced between two scalpel blades with a scissor-like action, while kept immersed in Medium 199 in a plastic petri dish. Small portions are then passed through a series of stainless steel sieves of graded pore diameter. The retaining mesh size depends on glomerular diameter and the optimal mesh for human and various animal glomeruli is detailed in Table 1.

The mince is gently pressed first through a 60-mesh (250μm) sieve with the back of a spoon or small beaker, while repeatedly washing with Medium 199 and 1% FCS to minimize adherence to any surface. The material passing through the mesh is collected in a petri dish, and the process is continued until only white connective tissue remains on the top of the mesh. The undersurface is then washed with jets of medium from a Pasteur pipette or syringe. The tissue fragments which have passed through this mesh are then pipetted through a series of meshes of gradually decreasing pore diameter. Successive meshes retain tubules and large tissue fragments until a mesh is reached which retains whole glomeruli and allows single cells and smaller glomerular fragments to pass through. Repeated washing over this last mesh allows a high degree of purity to be achieved, and this is checked frequently with a phase contrast microscope. The technique removes the parietal epithelial layer of Bowman's capsule during isolation in more than 80% of glomeruli. If tubular contamination remains as more than 2% of the total yield, further passage through all of the sieves is performed, or if single cells persist, further washing over the final sieve is undertaken. The final sieve for optimal glomerular yield and purity varies between species due to varying glomerular diameters; suitable pore size of sieves is indicated in Table 1. Improvements in technique include the use of nylon[19-21] rather than the traditional stainless steel for meshes, the maintenance of the tissue at around 4°C with ice, the use of siliconized glassware, and avoidance of overloading the meshes.[19]

**B. Glomerular Isolation by Microdissection**

Renal biopsy segments and other small pieces of tissue are examined by microdissection under a dissecting microscope. The segment is immersed in Medium 199 with 1% FCS and the glomeruli are teased out of the surrounding tissue using two 25-gauge needles on 1-mℓ syringes as handles. The glomeruli are then taken up with a 10-$\mu$ℓ pipette using a dissecting microscope, deposited in drops in a petri dish, and checked for purity. Contaminating tubules or cells are removed by diluting these drops and again picking off the isolated glomeruli, until 100% purity is attained as determined by phase microscopy.

**C. Glomerular Isolation Using Iron Infusion**

Although sieving techniques give satisfactory results for most species, isolation of glomeruli from rabbit kidneys using this method is tedious and often heavily contaminated with tubular fragments. A modification of the method of Cook and Pickering[22] whereby the kidneys are infused with iron and the iron-filled glomeruli are collected with a magnet, gives excellent results and like sieving takes less than an hour once mastered.

The rabbit is anesthetized with Nembutal (90 mg/kg) and given 1000 units of heparin via the marginal ear vein. The abdomen is aseptically opened, the kidney of each side grasped and reflected anteromedially, and the renal artery of each kidney cannulated with a 21-gauge butterfly needle. The artery is clamped or tied proximal to the needle and the kidney flushed with 50 mℓ of ice-cold saline.

A further 50 mℓ of 2 mg% $Fe_2O_3$ in saline is used to perfuse the kidney at a pressure of 120 mmHg, until the kidney begins to darken and swell; the kidneys are then removed, minced as before, and passed through a 100-gauge mesh to disrupt the kidney, and washed over a 300-gauge mesh to remove free iron particles. The glomeruli are then allowed to sediment while a magnet is held parallel to the beaker; iron-filled glomeruli are pulled laterally and other tissue and cells sink to the bottom and are aspirated. This is repeated several times until observation under a phase microscope shows pure glomeruli. Overinfusion of iron, giving jet black kidneys, results in considerable contamination of afferent arterioles, but this can often be eliminated by simple sieving.

**D Glomerular Isolation Using Ficoll Gradient**

An alternative method of glomerular isolation giving excellent yield and preservation of structure is that developed by Nørgaard.[18] This method involves renal perfusion with a cold salt solution to remove entrapped erythrocytes, then initial renal cortical disruption over a 250-$\mu$m sieve, followed by repeated washings of homogenate by centrifugation and resuspension, and then centrifugation over a discontinous Ficoll gradient. This centrifugation, which in effect acts as a viscosity gradient, results in the compact glomeruli migrating up through the layers, with a final purity of around 98% in the upper interphase. The glomeruli are further washed to remove the Ficoll and placed in culture.

In one of the few correlative studies[18] using light and electron microscopy (EM), glomeruli isolated by this method showed overall only minor changes compared with normal glomeruli. The disadvantages of the method include the need for satisfactory perfusion technique in vivo (which also renders isolation of human glomeruli difficult) and the need to avoid overloading the gradient since this markedly reduces the purity and yield. The latter limitation results in large numbers of gradient tubes being used if a large number of glomeruli are required.

## V. MORPHOLOGY OF ISOLATED GLOMERULI

Freshly isolated glomeruli may be examined morphologically by four techniques to ensure intact glomeruli with minimal structural disruption.

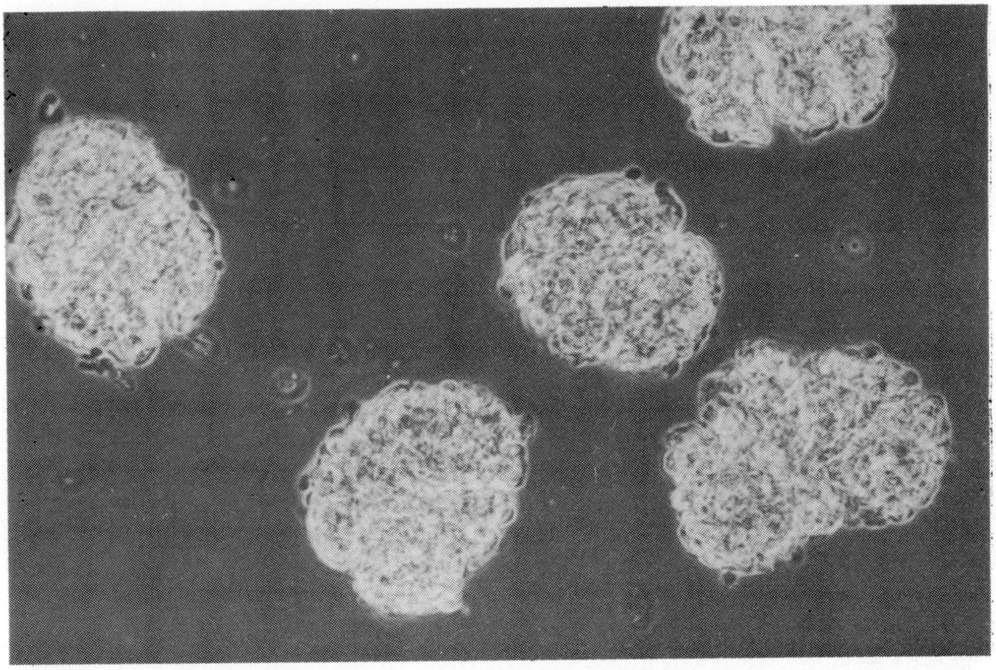

FIGURE 1. Isolated glomeruli illustrating purity of sample with absence of Bowman's capsule. (Phase contrast micrograph × 450 shown at 85%.)

1. Phase-contrast microscopy: During and after isolation procedure the glomeruli are viewed with phase contrast microscopy to confirm purity of the isolated glomeruli (Figure 1).
2. Light microscopy: Aliquots of glomeruli are fixed with Duboscq-Brasil, embedded in paraffin, and sections are cut at 2 μm thickness and stained with hematoxylin and eosin (HE), periodic acid Schiff reagent (PAS), and the periodic silver methenamine method.
3. Scanning EM: Glomeruli are fixed in 2.5% glutaraldehyde in 0.2 *M* cacodylate buffer (pH 7.4) and then washed with 0.1 *M* cacodylate buffer for at least 2 hr at room temperature and dehydrated through alcohols. Glomeruli are then critical-point dried, transferred to a stud, gold coated, and viewed in a scanning electron microscope.
4. Transmission EM: Glomeruli are fixed in 2.5% glutaraldehyde in 0.2 *M* cacodylate buffer (pH 7.4) overnight at 4°C. The glomeruli are then centrifuged at 1000 rpm for 5 min and the pellet post-fixed with 2% osmium tetroxide, and embedded in EPON or ARALDITE. Ultrathin (silver) sections are cut, stained with uranyl acetate and lead citrate, and viewed in a transmission electron microscope.

Glomeruli isolated by the above technique[6] show a uniform appearance on light microscopy of capillary loops supported by mesangial cells and matrix, lined by endothelial cells, and covered by visceral epithelial cells. Normal podocytic branching and interdigitations can be observed on transmission scanning EM with intact basement membrane and normal ultrastructure of all three cell types. Occasional myelin bodies in the podocyte cytoplasm occurred after 24 hr and after iron infusion of rabbit glomeruli, iron is seen lodged in the subendothelial spaces[23] as well as capillaries (Plate 6),* although the

* Plate 6 appears following page 88.

basement membrane remains intact. Other studies have confirmed essentially intact metabolic functions after these isolation techniques.[24-26]

## VI. TISSUE CULTURE OF ISOLATED GLOMERULI

**Vessels** — Vessels for glomerular culture include Rose chambers (after Rose),[27] cover slips in petri dishes, and tissue culture flasks such as Falcon flasks or Tissue Tek chamber/culture slides and flaskettes. We routinely use Falcon flasks (30 mℓ) because of their combination of good optical qualities and size, allowing simultaneous cultivation of many glomeruli with ease of handling.

**Physical and nutritional requirements** — These have been studied in detail;[6] various media including Medium 199, Eagles's minimum essential medium (MEM), and Ham's medium showed little difference in effect on glomerular culture, optimal temperature is 37°C, and optimal pH 7.4 with buffering best provided by Hepes buffer 20 m*M* and 0.03% sodium bicarbonate. Similarly, maximal attachment and growth rates occur using medium with 20% FCS added; batches of FCS and the tissue culture flasks vary and it is important that only samples from the same batch be used in a series of experiments. Finally, glomeruli require minimal movement during early culture to allow attachment and outgrowth to progress, and biweekly observation and medium change have been found most suitable. Penicillin (1000 units/mℓ) and streptomycin ( 100 $\mu$g/mℓ) are routinely added to medium.

**Technique** — Each Falcon flask is prepared by adding 7.5 mℓ of Medium 199 with 20% FCS, and up to 20 glomeruli per flask are added using a siliconized long Pasteur pipette. Tissue culture trays can also be used. Glomeruli in fewer numbers, such as from human renal biopsies, are cultured individually in drops. This method gives maximal attachment rates and avoids possible attachment in an optically useless flask corner or neck, and allows accurate determination of the origin of cell types in a given outgrowth.

For this method, a single glomerulus is pipetted into a 0.25-mℓ drop of medium in the center of the flask with 1 mℓ of medium along the flask rim to prevent dehydration. Up to three drops can be easily maintained per flask. Culturing of significantly more than 20 glomeruli per flask results in decreased attachment rates, although the cell growth of attached glomeruli is unaffected. In addition, the time spent in observation and counting of cell outgrowths of larger numbers of glomeruli results in protracted periods with the cultures at room temperature and changes in the growth pattern.

**Observation** — For the first week in culture most glomeruli remain floating freely in the medium, although some glomeruli begin to attach to the flask base by day 3. Attachment is assessed by gently rocking the flask and seeing whether the glomeruli remain firmly attached. From the time of attachment sequential observations of each glomerulus and its outgrowth are made using a phase contrast microscope with a calibrated vernier scale stage attachment. Analysis has shown that the number of glomeruli attaching with subsequent cellular outgrowth is independent of the method of isolation, sieving, or microdissection, and is similar for all species studied.[8]

Although the time of attachment of normal glomeruli varies from 3 to 14 days, the pattern of cells in the outgrowth is the same once attachment occurs with similar numbers of cells being present each day after attachment. Observations and counting of the cell types are usually performed twice weekly.

After about 2 weeks of cellular outgrowth, multilayering of cells and loss of differentiation tends to occur. Monolayering of cells over the whole flask surface is not seen with adult normal glomeruli in culture even after several months, unless addition of conditioned medium or culturing is undertaken or proteolytic enzymes such as trypsin or collagenase are used at the time of isolation.

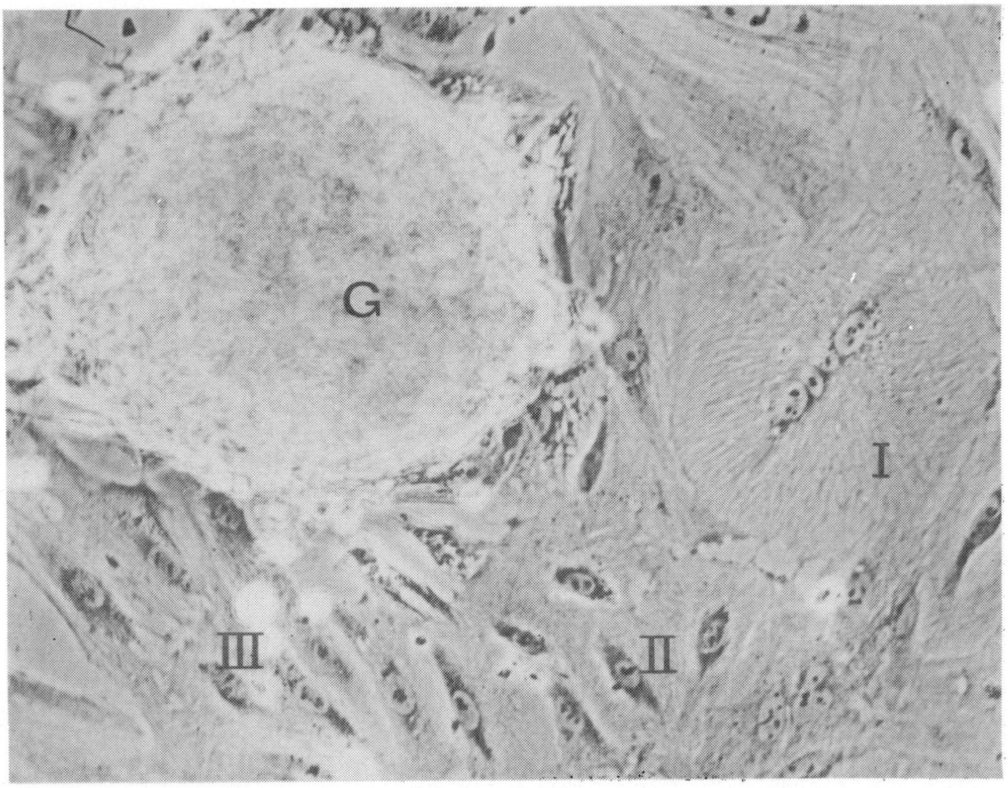


FIGURE 2. Phase contrast micrograph of glomerulus (G) in culture with the three cell types in outgrowth. (Magnification × 810.)

**Subculturing technique** — Isolation of single glomerular cells or subculturing of confluent glomerular outgrowths is performed by incubating in a 0.025% trypsin-0.5 m*M* disodium ethylenediaminetetracetic acid (EDTA) mixture in calcium-free and magnesium-free buffered salt soltuions (trypsin-versene), for 5 min at 37°C. Cells are resuspended at 100 mℓ for cloning, whereby 10-μℓ aliquots are taken and cultured with addition of conditioned medium, or at 100,000/mℓ for culture of dissociated glomerular cells.

**Conditioned medium** — The growth of individual glomerular cells from dissociated glomeruli or explants or whole glomeruli is possible using conditioned medium and insulin.[21] Conditioned medium may also increase the proportion of normal glomeruli attaching and forming outgrowths.

Whole glomeruli or glomerular cells, following subculturing, are added to medium supplemented with $10^{-6}$ *M* insulin and an equal volume of conditioned medium. This is prepared by passage through a 0.22-μm filter of medium harvested from log phase growth confluent cells, such as other normal glomerular cell cultures.[21]

## VII. NORMAL HUMAN GLOMERULAR CELLS IN CULTURE

Under the conditions described, three morphologically distinct cell types are seen in the outgrowth of normal human glomeruli.[5,6] On the basis of time of appearance in the outgrowth, the two main cell types have been designated Type I and Type II (Figure 2). A third cell type, seen on average once in every three outgrowths of normal glomeruli,

**Table 2**
**CHARACTERISTICS OF NORMAL HUMAN GLOMERULAR CELL TYPES IN CULTURE**

| Cell Type | I | II | III |
|---|---|---|---|
| Size (μm) | 50—150 | 15—50 | 6—10 |
| Shape | Arborized | Fusiform | Round |
| Ultrastructure | Sparse organelles | Numerous organelles | Phagolysosomes |
| | | **Microfilamentous microvilli** | |
| Division (average per 100 cells/day) | 0.1 | 2.0 | 0 |
| Molitity (μm/hr) | 0 | 12.2 | 250 |
| Latex phagocytosis | Present | Present | Present |
| Yeast phagocytosis | Absent | Present | Present |
| SRBC phagocytosis | Absent | Absent | Present |
| $C_c$ and Fc receptors | Absent | Absent | Present |
| Lysosome characteristics | Negative | Negative | Positive |
| β-Glucuronidase, acid phosphatase, esterase | Negative | Negative | Positive |
| Antiactin immunofluorescence | Negative | Negative | Negative |
| Cell identification | Epithelial | Mesangial | Macrophage |

is designated Type III. The following description is of cell types from human glomeruli in culture but similar features apply to many other species.[11]

### A. Type I Cells

These are large stellate cells, maximal diameter 100 to 150 μm which appear during the first week of outgrowth. They are often multinucleate, averaging 1.7 ± 0.2 nuclei per cell (n = 200). Their complex cytoplasmic appearance, with primary, secondary, and tertiary branching, is lost over a variable period in culture; the branching cytoplasm tends to fuse peripherally leaving large circular cells with a "vacuolated" appearance. These cells display little motility and show contact inhibition. Their rate of division is 0.2 divisions per 100 cells/day of culture, and their maximal number in culture is found around 2 weeks. After this time numbers remain constant or decreased as occasional cells die (Table 2).

Scanning EM of glomerular cultures show these large Type I cells migrating from the capillary loop surface onto the culture flask and they are seen to have small villous processes (Figure 3). Ultrastructurally Type I cells have a sparse featureless cytoplasm with few granules (Figure 4). Type I cells are unable to phagocytose yeast or larger particles. They do not appear to have Fc or C3b receptors.

### B. Type II Cells

These are smaller than Type I cells, with a fusiform shape. They are usually 15 to 50 μm long. They have a dense, homogeneous cytoplasm, usually with a single nucleus. They are motile cells with gliding movements of up to 40 μm/hr. They do not demonstrate contact inhibition, tending to form layers after several weeks in culture, and also undergo dedifferentiation often to become larger divisions per 100 cells in culture per day, but accumulate at a rate of 30 cells per 100 cells per day of culture by emigration from the

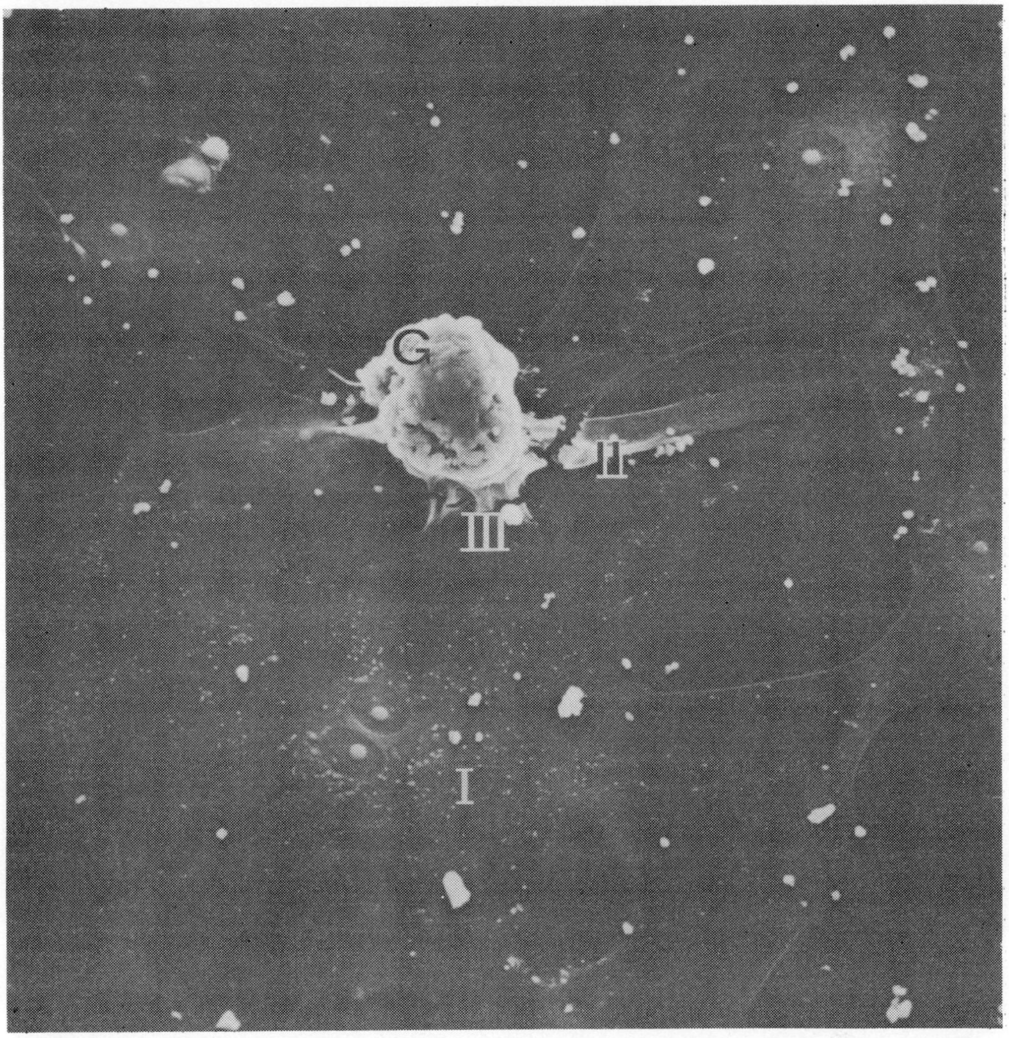


FIGURE 3. Scanning EM of glomerulus (G) and its outgrowth with multi-nucleated Type I cells, spindle-shaped Type II cells, and Type III cells. (Magnification × 765.)

glomerulus particularly after the first week. After the second week they are the predominant cells in the outgrowth (Table 2).

Scanning EM shows microvilli on Type II cells (Figure 3) and transmission EM (Figure 4) shows a prominent endoplasmic reticulum, numerous mitochondria, and a microfilamentous skeleton. They can ingest more avidly than Type I cells, and ingest yeast. They have no Fc or C3b receptors.

### C. Type III Cells

Found on average once in every three normal glomerular outgrowths, these cells are difficult to distinguish from dividing Type II cells unless cinemicroscopy is used. They are round, refractile cells with a diameter of 10 to 15 $\mu$m, though they occasionally spread on the flask to form cells up to 50 $\mu$m in diameter. Using cinemicroscopy they are immediately distinguished by their constant mobility (up to 300 $\mu$m/hr) and pseudopodia identical to those of peritoneal macrophages in culture. They tend to remain close to the glomerulus, often reentering then reappearing from the glomerulus (Table

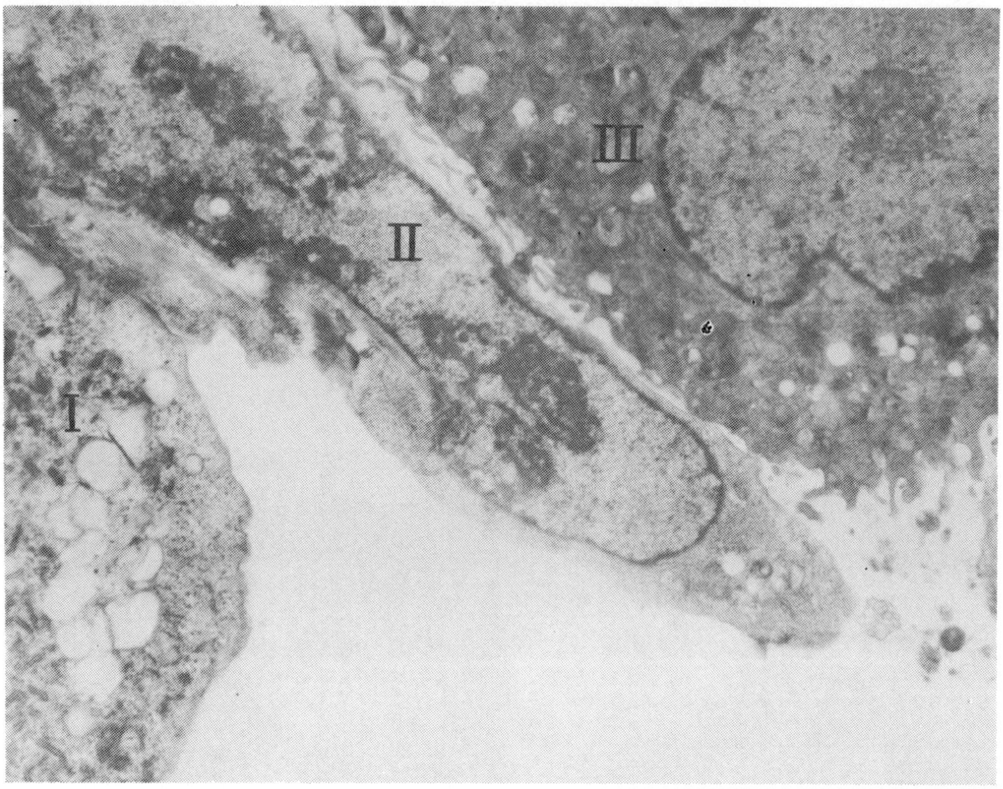


FIGURE 4. Transmission electron micrograph of Type I cell with sparse vacuolated bytoplasm, elongated dense Type II cell, and Type III cell with microvilli (macrophage). (Magnification × 3500.)

2). On scanning EM these Type III cells show microvilli, and transmission EM shows prominent phagolysosomes (Figure 5).

Further evidence for the identification of Type III cells as macrophages is provided by the presence of Fc and C3b receptors, their phagocytosis of cell debris, latex, yeast, and red blood cells, and their histochemical profile in staining strongly for β-glucuronidase, nonspecific esterase, and acid phosphatase.

Type III cells, thus demonstrated to be macrophages, probably emerge in culture from their intracapillary location by migrating across the basement membrane and/or from the vascular pole into the medium. The cells are very rarely seen in normal glomerular cultures. However, they represent the major cell in the glomerular outgrowths from patients and experimental animals with crescentic glomerulonephritis.[6,7,28-32] This observation incriminated the macrophage in crescent formation.[28]

## VIII. ANALYSIS OF GLOMERULAR OUTGROWTH

In addition to standard observation of glomerular outgrowths using phase-contrast microscopy, several additional techniques are needed.

### A. Transmission EM of Glomerular Outgrowths

The culture medium is renewed the evening before fixing. The following day the flask is rinsed twice with Hank's single strength medium at 37°C, and then fixed with cold 2.5% glutaraldehyde in 0.2 *M* cacodylate buffer, pH 7.4, for 24 hr and post-fixed in

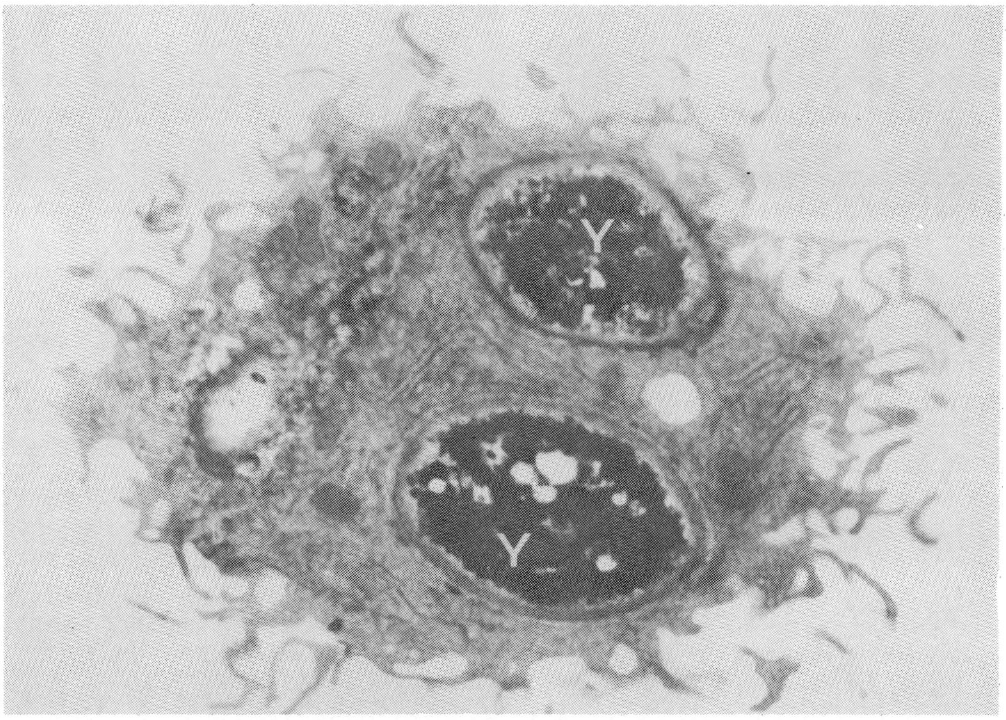


FIGURE 5. Transmission electron micrograph of cytoplasm of Type III cell (macrophage) demonstrating phagocytosis of yeast (Y). (Magnification × 13,700.)

osmium. The flask is then washed three times with cacodylate buffer for 30 min and again in uranyl acetate, dehydrated through 50, 70, and 90% cold alcohols, and transferred to cold absolute alcohol with two changes, for 1 hr at room temperature.

The flask neck and lid are cut off and EPON added to a depth of 2 mm. After 4 hr the flask is heated to 60°C for 10 min, the plastic drained, and fresh EPON added. After a further 4-hr period at room temperature, capsules filled with EPON are placed over the glomeruli which have been marked on the undersurface with a diamond marker. Polymerization for 24 hr at 60°C follows and then while warm, the capsules with adherent glomeruli and outgrowths are snapped off. Silver sections are cut on an ultramicrotome, stained with uranyl acetate and lead citrate, and viewed in a transmission electron microscope.

**B. Scanning EM of Glomerular Outgrowths**

The medium is renewed before fixation. Fixation with 2.5% glutaraldehyde in 0.2 *M* cacodylate for 24 hr at 4°C is performed, followed by rinsing three times with 0.1 *M* cacodylate and dehydration through alcohols. Critical point drying is performed, the specimen transferred to a stud, gold coating done using a sputter coater, and the section viewed in a scanning electron microscope (Figure 3).

**C. Phase-Contrast Cine Microscopy**

Using a phase-contrast microscope and a camera attachment, plus a thermostatic heated stage, glomerular outgrowths are followed during the period of their growth. Flasks are kept at 37°C and filmed at one frame per minute for 1 to 20 days. Phagocytosis (see below) is assessed by filming at one frame per 6 sec for 30 to 60 min. Resultant films are analyzed with a photo-optical data analyzer. An alternative approach with an added feature of "instant replay" is using the time-lapse camera and video-tape recorder.

**D. Assessment of Phagocytic Capacity**

Latex beads (1.2μm diameter) or Baker's yeast (4μm diameter) which has been opsonized by incubation with fresh human serum at 37°C for 1 hr is made up as 0.5% (V/V) suspension in saline. Two hundred microliters is added to a flask while filming at one frame per 6 sec and continued for 30 min at 37°C. The culture is then fixed for transmission EM as previously described.

Sheep erythrocytes in a 5% (V/V) suspension are sensitized with an equal volume of commercial hemolyser in a subhemagglutinating dose, incubated at 37°C for 30 min, washed three times with saline, and resuspended to 2% (V/V); 50 μℓ of this suspension is added to each flask and filming is continued at one frame per 6 sec for 1 hr. The hypotonic lysis is performed, using saline diluted 1:4 with distilled water for 15 sec and isotonicity is restored with fresh medium 199. Phagocytosis of erythrocytes is assessed using a phase-contrast microscope and the flask fixed for transmission EM.

**E. Fc and C3b Receptors**

Commercial rabbit antiserum to sheep erythrocytes (A) Hemolysin is fractionated to obtain IgG and IgM fractions, using G-200 Sephadex®. Each fraction is tested by hemagglutinin against sheep erythrocytes (E) which have been stored in Alsever's solution for 1 or 2 weeks, washed four times in phosphate buffered saline (PBS) (200 g, 10 min), and resuspended to $1 \times 10^9$ cells per mℓ (~ 5% V/V). The minimal subagglutinating dilution of antiserum is then used to sensitize sheep erythrocytes (EA), by incubating equal volumes of 5% cells and IgG or IgM for 30 min at 37°C.

Fc receptors are detected by washing the sensitized erythrocytes (IgG-EA) (200 g for 10 min) three times in PBS, and resuspending to 0.25% (V/V) and adding 3 mℓ of this indicator to each Falcon falsk which has been drained of medium. After 30 min at room temperature the flask is rinsed three times with phosphate buffered saline (PBS) to remove nonadherent erythrocytes, and the glomeruli examined under the phase microscope and photographed, and fixed for scanning EM. Negative control for the test is unsensitized sheep erythrocytes (E) and the positive control is the flask of macrophages in culture.[38]

C3b receptors are detected by first preparing IgM-EA 2.5% (V/V), washing three times (220 g, 10 min) with veronal buffered saline (VBS) at 4°C and adding an equal volume of freshly drawn human serum diluted 1:4 or guinea-pig serum diluted 1:50, the resultant IgM-EAC suspension being incubated at 4°C for 30 min, washed three times (200 g, 10 min) with VBS at 4°C, resuspended to 0.25% (V/V) and added to the Falcon flask for 1 hr at room temperature, and then for 1 hr at 4°C. Nonadherent erythrocytes are removed by washing three times with ice-cold VBS and the outgrowth examined with phase microscopy. The flask with outgrowth is then fixed for scanning EM as previously described. Controls for this experiment include IgM-EA and macrophages[38] in culture.

**F. Histochemistry of Glomerular Cells in Culture**

As an extension of previous work,[33] the enzymes found particularly useful in characterizing cells of the monocyte-macrophage line, β-glucuronidase, acid phosphatase, and sodium fluoride-sensitive esterase, have been sought in glomerular cells in culture. β-Glucuronidase is not found in the normal glomerulus and those enzymes mentioned are only in trace amounts. All three enzymes are strongly positive in Type III cells, with β-glucuronidase found only in Type III cells.

The techniques used to demonstrate enzyme activity are based on the formation of azo dyes; naphthol-conjugated substances are incubated with the tissue, and, if the enzyme is present, free naphthol is liberated and combines with a diazonium salt in the medium to form a colored azo dye. The dye formation, therefore, allows semiquantitation of the amount of enzyme present. Negative controls include incubation in the absence of substrate and in the presence of the specific inhibitor of the enzyme being tested, and positive control is a flask of macrophages in culture.[38] For each enzyme, incubation without fixation results in the greatest intensity of staining and a range of incubation times is used, with over-long incubations resulting in diffusion of dye and secondary nonspecific labeling of other cells in culture.

**β-Glucuronidase** — The substrate and diazonium salt are prepared by the method of Hayashi.[33] The glomerular outgrowth is rinsed with fresh medium added to the flask. The incubation occurs at 37°C and optimal staining occurs at 2 to 3 hr. The incubation medium is removed, the flask rinsed with medium, and the outgrowth examined under the phase microscope. Precipitates in the medium can be avoided by incubating the outgrowths upside down or by replacing the incubation medium with fresh incubation medium warmed to 37°C each hour. The specific inhibitor of this enzyme is 1,4-saccharolactone ($10^{-4}$ *M*, adding 2 mg/100 mℓ). Presence of the enzyme is indicated by a bright red reaction product (Plate 7).*

**Acid phosphatase** — The substrate and diazonium salt are prepared as described by Barka and Anderson.[34] The technique is as for β-glucuronidase with incubation at 37°C for 15-min intervals to 1 hr. The specific inhibitor is sodium fluoride ($10^{-2}$ *M*), and a positive reaction is indicated by a brick red color.

**Sodium fluoride-sensitive esterase** — This type of esterase is found only in cells of the monocyte-macrophage series and not in other phagocytic cells such as polymorphonuclear leucocytes.[35] The reagents are prepared by the method of Pearse,[36] and the method is as described for β-glucuronidase, except that incubation occurs at room temperature, and $10^{-2}$ *M* sodium fluoride is the specific inhibitor. Again a brick red color indicates the enzyme's presence.

### G. Detection of Antigens on Glomerular Cells in Culture by Rosetting

Cell surface antigens of glomerular cells in culture may be detected using antibody-coated sheep red blood cells (SRBC). The antigen may be recognized by a specific antibody coupled to the SRBC or by an indirect method in incubation with antiserum and then incubated with heterologous anti-Ig antibody coupled with SRBC may be used. The technique has the features of sensitivity, quantitation, and reproducibility compared to immunofluorescence, and speed compared to autoradiography.

The antibody is coupled to the SRBC as described by Parish and McKenzie,[37] using $CrCl_3$. The flasks containing the glomerular outgrowths are rinsed twice with saline and antibody-coated SRBC in PBS with 10% FCS are added over the outgrowth which has been previously circled with a diamond marker on the flask under surface. The flask and antibody-coated red cells are centrifuged at 200 g for 5 min to allow close opposition of cells and outgrowth, and incubated at 4°C for 30 min. The flask is then rinsed three times with PBS and 1% FCS and examined under a phase-contrast microscope (direct method) and then similarly incubated with second label (indirect method) washed and examined. Type II cells are labeled in this way and clusters of red cells may be seen adherent to them (Figure 6). The indirect method, allowing simultaneous testing of multiple antisera, is preferred because of its convenience; the second label used is a heterologous anti-Ig antiserum. Thus rabbit anti-mouse Ig (RAM) is coupled to SRBC, and optimal rosetting with minimal aggregation is determined using mouse spleen cells. This is necessary because the amount of $CrCl_3$ required for optimal coupling varies with too much $CrCl_3$ causing clumping of SRBC and too little resulting in poor rosette formation.

* Plate 7 appears following page 88.

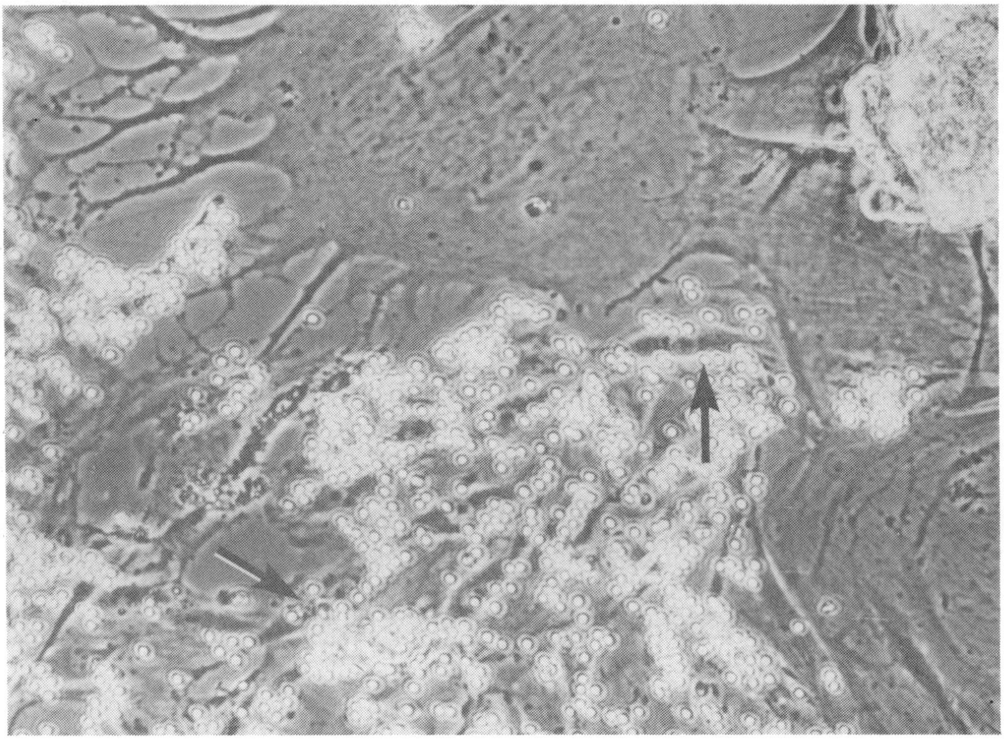

FIGURE 6. Identification of Type II cells by rosetting on them (arrows) of sensitized sheep red blood cells. Other Type II cells are completely obscured by dense labeling. (Phase contrast micrograph × 450.)

Controls for these experiments include a nonspecific protein coupled to SRBC such as bovine serum albumin (for direct method) and incubated with normal serum, or PBS and 10% FCS instead of first antibody (for indirect method); all outgrowths in a given experiment should be from normal tissue and cultured under the same conditions and for the same duration. Multiple antisera are conveniently tested after culturing individual glomeruli in 96 well trays, and treating these as described for flasks.

**H. Detection of Antigens on Glomerular Cells in Culture by Autoradiography**

Antigens of glomerular cells in culture may be detected using autoradiography. The cells are cultured in Lab-Tek slide culture chambers washed twice with saline and incubated with antiserum for 1 hr at room temperature. The cells are then washed for 15 min with three changes of PBS and 1% FCS on a horizontal shaker at a standard speed of 30 horizontal excursions per minute. The buffer is drained and a second incubation with heterologous anti-Ig antibody coupled to $I^{125}$ follows, again for 1 hr at room temperature. The cells are washed and then fixed with the addition of 2.5% glutaraldehyde in PBS for 5 min. The cells are rinsed and allowed to dry and the plastic casing removed from the slides.

After drying, the slides are dipped in Ilford emulsion G4, diluted 1:2 with distilled water at 45°C in a dark room; they are dried overnight at room temperature and then exposed to 4°C in silica gel containing light-tight boxes. Suitable intervals for exposure are determined by dipping multiple slides and developing sample slides at intervals.

The slides are developed in the dark by placing in Kodak® D-19 developer for 3 min, then in 1% acetone for 1 min followed by 3 min in Rapid fixer. They are then washed in distilled water, no longer in the darkroom, for 1 hr, stained with toluidine blue, mounted in Depex, and examined (Figure 7).

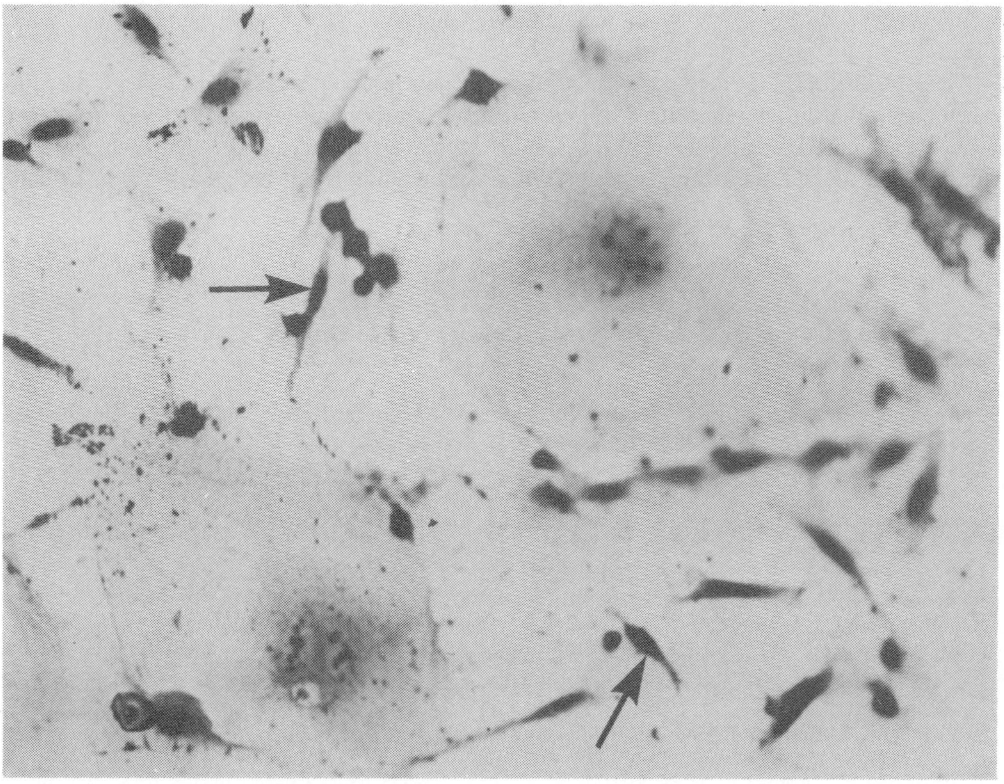

FIGURE 7. Type I and Type II cells from glomerular culture outgrowth, seen with labeling of Type II cells by an indirect autoradiographic method (arrows). (Magnification of × 400.)

Controls include incubation with normal serum instead of antiserum and slides without incubation with $I^{125}$ (positive chemotherapy) and exposed to light after dipping in emulsion (negative chemotherapy).

## I. Immunofluorescence of Glomerular Cells in Culture

Cells are cultured in the standard manner in Falcon flasks or slide culture/chambers and washed with PBS and 1% FCS for 5 min at a standard speed of 30 horizontal excursions per minute. The PBS is drained and cells covered with the antiserum after marking the area on the back of the flask or slide with a diamond marker. The antiserum is incubated with the cells for 30 min at room temperature and is then washed off using three washes of PBS and 1% FCS for 5 min each at the standard shaker speed. The cells are drained and then treated with a FITC-labeled heterologous anti-Ig for 30 min at room temperature. The cells are finally washed as for the first antiserum and mounted in buffered glycerol (pH 8.6 — i.e., glycerol in PBS V/V) and examined by UV and narrow-band fluorescence microscopy immediately.

Antibody activity against cell membrane antigens is titrated with serial dilutions of test sera, and controls include incubation with normal serum and conjugate. Nonspecific staining may require absorption with homologous tissues such as liver. Fixation of cells is best avoided, and the effects of any fixative which is used should be evaluated carefully beforehand. Capping or endocytosis of bound antibody may occur, but can be avoided by incubation at 4°C or in the presence of sodium azide (0.01%) with azide being omitted in the last wash, followed by immediate examination.

## IX. SUMMARY

The culture of isolated glomeruli provides a new method of appraisal of glomerular pathology. Techniques of filtration and culture have been described for both man and other species. Modifications of many standard techniques, including light, EM, and cine microscopy, as well as methods for examination of glomerular cell markers, have been described.

## REFERENCES

1. **Bernick, M. B.,** Contractile activity of human glomeruli in culture, *Nephron,* 6, 1, 1969.
2. **Quadracci, L. J. and Striker, G. E.,** Growth and maintenance of glomerular cells in vitro, *Proc. Soc. Exp. Biol. Med.,* 135, 947, 1970.
3. **Burlington, H. and Cronkite, E. P.,** Characteristics of cell cultures derived from renal glomeruli, *Proc. Soc. Exp. Biol. Med.,* 142, 143, 1973.
4. **Atkins, R. C., Glasgow, E., and Mathews, F.,** The culture of isolated glomeruli, *Aust. N. Z. J. Med.,* 4, 427, 1974.
5. **Holdsworth, S. R., Glasgow, E. F., Thomson, N. M., and Atkins, R. C.,** Normal human glomerular cells in culture, *J. Pathol.,* 126, 231, 1978.
6. **Holdsworth, S. R., Glasgow, E. F., Thomson, N. M., and Atkins, R. C.,** Tissue culture of isolated human glomeruli, *Pathology,* 10, 59, 1978.
7. **Atkins, R. C., Glasgow, E. F., Holdsworth, S. R., Thomson, N. M., and Hancock, W. W.,** Tissue culture of isolated glomeruli from patients with glomerulonephritis, *Kidney Int.,* 17, 515, 1980.
8. **Holdsworth, S. R.,** The Tissue Culture of Normal and Diseased Isolated Glomeruli, thesis, Monash University, 1978.
9. **Fish, A. J., Michael, A. F., Vernier, R. L., and Brown, D. M.,** Human glomerular cells in tissue culture, *Lab. Invest.,* 33, 330, 1975.
10. **Oberley, T. D., Burkholder, P. M., Barber, T. A., and Hwang, C.,** Cytochemical characteristics of cultured adult guinea pig glomerular cells, *Invest. Cell Pathol.,* 2, 27, 1979.
11. **Holdsworth, S. R., Glasgow, E. F., Atkins, R. C., and Thomson, N. M.,** Cell characteristics of cultured glomeruli from different species, *Nephron,* 22, 4, 454, 1978.
12. **Paul, J. R.,** *Cells and Tissue Culture,* 4th ed., Livingston, Edinburgh, 1970.
13. **Kruse, P. F. and Patterson, M. K.,** *Tissue Culture and Applications,* Academic Press, New York, 1974.
14. **Greenspon, S. A. and Krakower, C. A.,** Direct evidence for the antigenicity of the glomeruli in the production of nephrotoxic serum, *Arch. Pathol.,* 49, 291, 1950.
15. **Krakower, C. A. and Greenspon, S. A.,** Localization of the nephrotoxic antigen within the isolated renal glomerulus, *Arch. Pathol.,* 51, 629, 1951.
16. **Fong, J. S. C. and Drummond, K. N.,** Method of preparation of glomeruli for metabolic studies, *J. Lab. Clin. Med.,* 71, 1034, 1968.
17. **Portis, J. L., Wikel, S. K., and McAtee, F. J.,** A simplified rapid method for purification of glomeruli, *J. Clin. Pathol.,* 32, 406, 1979.
18. **Nørgaard, J. O. R.,** A new method for the isolation of ultra structurally preserved glomeruli, *Kidney Int.,* 9, 278, 1976.
19. **Misra, R. P.,** Isolation of glomeruli from mammalian kidneys by graded sieving, *Am. J. Clin. Pathol.,* 58, 135, 1972.
20. **Burkholder, P. M., Oberley, T. D., Barber, T. A., Beacom, A., and Koehler, C.,** Immune adherence in renal glomeruli; complement receptor sites on glomerular capillary epithelial cells, *Am. J. Pathol.,* 86, 635, 1977.
21. **Oberley, T. D., Burkholder, P. M., and Mills, M. D.,** Culture of human glomerular cells, *Am. J. Pathol.,* 96, 101, 1979.
22. **Cook, W. F. and Pickering, G. W.,** A rapid method for separating glomeruli from rabbit kidney, *Nature,* 182, 1103, 1958.
23. **Meezan, E., Brendel, K., Ulreich, J., and Carlson, E.,** Properties of a pure metabolically active glomerular preparation from rat kidneys. I. Isolation, *J. Pharmacol. Exp. Ther.,* 187, 332, 1973.
24. **Taylor, G. G., Price, R. G., and Franz, H. E.,** The distribution of some hydrolases in glomeruli and tubular fragments prepared from rat kidney by zonal centrifugation, *Biochem. J.,* 122, 641, 1971.
25. **Krisko, I. and Walker, W. G.,** Protein and glycoprotein synthesis by isolated kidney glomeruli, *Proc. Soc. Exp. Biol. Med.,* 146, 942, 1974.

26. **Brendal, K. and Meezan, E.,** Properties of a pure metabolically active glomerular preparation from rat kidneys. II. Metabolism, *J. Pharmacol. Exp. Ther.,* 187, 342, 1973.
27. **Rose, G.,** The circumfusion system for multipurpose culture chambers. I. Introduction to the mechanics, techniques and basic results of a 12 chamber (in vitro) closed circulation system, *J. Cell Biol.,* 32, 89, 1967.
28. **Atkins, R. C., Holdsworth, S. R., Glasgow, E. F., and Mathews, F. E.,** The macrophage in human rapidly progressive glomerulonephritis, *Lancet,* 1, 830, 1976.
29. **Holdsworth, S. R., Thomson, N. M., Glasgow, E. F., Dowling, J. P., and Atkins, R. C.,** Tissue culture of isolated glomeruli in experimental crescentic glomerulonephritis, *J. Exp. Med.,* 147, 98, 1978.
30. **Holdsworth, S. R., Allen, D., Thomson, N. M., Glasgow, E. F., and Atkins, R. C.,** Histochemistry of glomerular cells in animal models of glomerulonephritis, *Pathology,* 12, 339, 1980.
31. **Thomson, N. M., Holdsworth, S. R., Glasgow, E. F., and Atkins, R. C.,** The macrophage in the development of experimental crescentic glomerulonephritis; studies using tissue culture and electron microscopy, *Am. J. Pathol.,* 94, 223, 1979.
32. **Holdsworth, S. R., Thomson, N. M., Glasgow, E. F., and Atkins, R. C.,** The effect of defribination on macrophage participation in rabbit nephrotoxic nephritis: studies using glomerular culture and electron microscopy, *Clin. Exp. Immunol.,* 37, 28, 1979.
33. **Hayashi, M., Nakajima, Y., and Fishman, W. H.,** The cytologic demonstration of a δ-glucuronidase employing naphthol AS-RI glucuronide and hexazonium pararosaniline, *J. Histochem. Cytochem.,* 12, 293, 1964.
34. **Barka, T. and Anderson, P. J.,** Histochemical methods for acid phosphatase using hexazonium pararosaniline as coupler, *J. Histochem. Cytochem.,* 10, 741, 1962.
35. **Braunsteiner, H. and Schmalzl, F.,** Cytochemistry of monocytes and macrophages, *Mononuclear Phagocytes,* Van Furth, R., Ed., Blackwell, Oxford, 1970, chap. 5.
36. **Pearse, A. G. E.,** *Histochemistry: Theoretical and Applied,* Vol. 2, Churchill Livingston, London, 1972, 1303.
37. **Parish, C. R. and McKenzie, I. F. C.,** A sensitive rosetting method for detecting subpopulations of lymphocytes which react with all alloantisera, *J. Immunol. Methods,* 20, 173, 1978.
38. **Stuart, A. E., Habeshaw, J. A., and Davidson, A. E.,** Phagocytes in vitro, in *Handbook of Experimental Immunology,* 3rd. ed., Weir, D. M., Blackwell, Oxford, 1978, 31.4.
39. **Atkins, R. C., Glasgow, E. F., Holdsworth, S. R., and Thomson, N. M.,** Glomerular cells in glomerulonephritis, in *Progress in Glomerulonephritis,* Kincaid-Smith, P., d'Apice, A., and Atkins, R. C., Eds., John Wiley & Sons, New York, 1979, 91.

# APPENDIX

## EQUIPMENT SUPPLIERS LIST

Since there are many suppliers of specialist equipment in most countries, it is impractical to attempt to provide a comprehensive listing. Instead we have listed major manufacturers and suppliers in several countries. Enquiries to these addresses may reveal a local source of supply.

### General Laboratory Chemicals

Calbiochem
10933 North Torrey Pines Road
La Jolla, Calif. 92037

Eastman Kodak Co.
Rochester, N.Y. 14650

Fisher Scientific Co.
633 Greenwich Street
New York, N.Y. 10014

Polysciences Inc.
Paul Valley Industrial Park
Warrington, Pa. 18796

British Drug Houses Ltd.
Poole
Dorset, BH 12 4NN
England

Hopkins and Williams Ltd.
Chadwell Heath
Essex RM1 1HA
England

May and Baker Ltd.
Dagenham
Essex RM10 7XS
England

Fluka AG.
Chemische Fabrik
Buchs SG
Switzerland

E. Merck
61 Dormstadt
West Germany

May and Baker Australia Pty. Ltd.
715 Elizabeth Street
Waterloo
N.S.W. 2118
Australia

B.D.H. (Aust) Ltd.
P.O. Box 168
Boronia, Victoria, 3155
Australia

### General Laboratory Apparatus

Fisher Scientific Co.
633 Greenwich Street
New York, N.Y. 10014

Ladd Research Industries, Inc.
P.O. Box 901
Burlington, Vt. 05401

Baird and Tatlock
P.O. Box 1
Romford RM1 HA
Essex
England

Jencons (Scientific) Ltd.
Mark Road
Hemel Hempstead
Hertfordshire
England

Ramsay Surgical Ltd.
182 Berkley Street
Carlton
Victoria 3053
Australia

Selby Scientific Ltd.
352 Ferntree Gully Road
Notting Hill 3168
Australia

### Disposable Laboratory Apparatus

Ladd Research Industries Ind.
P.O. Box 901
Burlington, Vt. 05401

Camlab Ltd.
Nuffield Road
Cambridge CB4 1TH
England

Disposable Products Pty. Ltd.
22 Barongarook Count
Lower Plenty
Victoria 3093
Australia

### Specialist Materials for Optical and EM Stains

Polysciences Inc.
Paul Valley Industrial Park
Warrington, Pa. 19876

Difco Laboratories (UK)
P.O. Box 14B
Central Avenue
West Molesey
Surrey
England

G. T. Gurr
Searle Scientific Services
Coronation Road
Cressex Industrial Estate
Buckinghamshire
England

Selby Scientific Ltd.
352 Ferntree Gully Road
Notting Hill
Victoria 3168
Australia

Ramsay Surgical Ltd.
182 Berkley Street
Carlton
Victoria, 33
Australia

### Embedding Materials

Ciba Co. Inc.
Plastics Division
Kimberton, Pa. 19442

Miles Laboratories Ind.
P.O. Box 2000
Elkart, Ind. 46515

Polysciences Inc.
Paul Valley Industrial Park
Warrington, Pa. 18976

Ciba-Geigy
Duxford
Cambridge
England

Fluka (U.K. agents)
Fluorochem
Dinting Lane
Glossop
Derbyshire SK13 9NU
England

Fluka AG.
Chemische Fabrik
Buchs SG.
Switzerland

Gelman Clemco Pty. Ltd.
1 Princess Street
Kew
Victoria 3101
Australia

## Embedding Materials (continued)

Miles Laboratories Aust. Pty. Ltd.
Wellington Road
Mulgrave
Victoria 3170
Australia

Ramsay Surgical Ltd.
182 Berkley Street
Carlton
Victoria 3053
Australia

Selby Scientific Ltd.
352 Ferntree Gully Road
Notting Hill
Victoria 3053
Australia

## Microtomes, Ultramicrotomes, and Glass Knife Makers

Du Pont Co.
Industrial Products Division
Sorvall Operations
Newton, Conn. 06470

E. Leitz Co.
468 Park Avenue South
New York, N.Y. 10016

E. Leitz Instruments Ltd.
30 Mortimer Street
London W1
England

LKB Instruments Ltd.
232 Addington Road
South Croydon CR2 8YD
Surrey
England

LKB-Producer AB
S-161 25 Bromma
Sweden

C. Reichert Ltd.
Hernalser Hauptstrasse 219
A-1171
Wein
Austria

LKB (Australian agents)
Linbrook Int.
Park Street
South Melbourne
Victoria
Australia

Reichert (Australian agents)
Selby Scientific Ltd.
352 Ferntree Gully Road
Notting Hill, 3168
Australia

## Cryostats

Miles Laboratories Inc.
P.O. Box 2000
Elkart, Ind. 46515

Slee
179 Lanier Road
Hither Green Lane
London SE13 6Qd
England

Miles Laboratories Australia Pty. Ltd.
Wellington Road
Mulgrave
Victoria 3170
Australia

**Automatic Processing Machines**

Fisher Scientific Co.
633 Greenwich Street
New York, N.Y. 10014

Miles Laboratories Inc.
P.O. Box 2000
Elkart Ind. 46515

C. Reichert Ltd.
Hernalser Hauptstrasse 219
A-1171
Wein
Austria

Sakura Finetechnical Co. Ltd.
9 Honcho 3 Chome
Tokyo 103
Japan

Fisher Scientific and Sakura
(Australian agents)
Ramsay Surgical Ltd.
183 Berkley Street
Carlton
Victoria 3053
Australia

Miles Laboratories Australia Pty. Ltd.
Wellington Road
Mulgrave
Victoria, 3170
Australia

Reichert (Australian agents)
Selby Scientific Ltd.
352 Ferntree Gully Road
Notting Hill 3168
Australia

**EM Laboratory Tools and Equipment, EM Fixation Chemicals**

Ernest F. Fullam Inc.
P.O. Box 444
Schenectady, N.Y. 12301

Du Pont (Diamond Knives)
Wilmington, Del. 19898

Ladd Research Industries Ind.
P.O. Box 901
Burlington, Vt. 05401

Polysciences Inc.
Paul Valley Industrial Park
Warrington, Pa. 18976

Taab (U.S.A. agents)
Ebtec Corp.
120 Shoemaker Lane
Agawam, Mass. 01001

Du Pont (Diamond Knives)
Wilbury House
Hitchin
Hertfordshire
England

Polaron Equipment Ltd.
60/62 Greenhill Crescent
Holywell Estates
Watford
Hertfordshire
England

Taab Laboratories
40 Grovelands Road
Reading
Berkshire
England

Balzers Union AG
Postfach 75
FL-9496 Balzers
Furstentum
Liechtenstein

Du Pont de Nemours S.A.
(Diamond Knives)
9 Rue de Vienne
Paris 8
France

Polaron (Australian agents)
Selby Scientific Ltd.
352 Ferntree Gully Road
Notting Hill 3168
Australia

Taab (Australian agents)
Lab Supply Pty. Ltd.
37-39 Woodlands Terrace
Edwardstown S.A. 5031
Australia

Polysciences (Australian agents)
John Morris Aust. Pty. Ltd.
P.O. Box 80
Chatswood
N.S.W. 2067
Australia

**Photographic Materials**

Eastman Kodak Co.
Rochester, N.Y. 14650

Ilford Ltd. (U.S.A. agency)
Polysciences Inc.
Paul Valley Industrial Park
Warrington, Pa. 18976

Ilford Ltd.
Southern Distribution Centre
Christopher Martin Road
Basildon
Essex
England

Kodak Ltd.
P.O. Box 33
Swallowdale Lane
Hemel Hempstead
Hertfordshire HP2 7EU
England

Ilford Foto B.V.
Jan Rebelstraat 5
Amsterdam
The Netherlands

Kodak-Nederland B.V.
Zeisterweg 1
Odijk
The Netherlands

Ilford Australia Pty. Ltd.
Ferntree Gully Road
Notting Hill
Victoria, 3168
Australia

Kodak (A'Asia) Pty. Ltd.
173 Elizabeth Street
Coburg
Victoria, 3058
Australia

**Immunochemicals**

Calbiochem
10933 North Torrey Pines Road
La Jolla, Calif. 92037

Dakopatts, (U.S.A. agents)
Accurate Chemical and Scientific Corp.
28 Tech Street
Hicksville, N.Y. 11801

Miles Laboratories Inc.
P.O. Box 2000
Elkart, Ind. 46515

Dakopatts (British agents)
Mercia Diagnostics Ltd.
Paramount Industrial Estate
Sandown Road
Watford WD2 4XA
England

**Immunochemicals (continued)**

Wellcome Reagents Ltd.
Beckenham
Kent BR3 3BS
England

Dakopatts A/S
Guldborgvej 22
Postbox 1404
2000 Copenhagen F
Denmark

Dakopatts, (Australian agents)
Bio-Scientific
118 North West Arm Road
Gymnea N.S.W. 2227
Australia

Calbiochem-Behring (Aust) Pty. Ltd.
382 Whitehorse Road
Nunawading 3131
Australia

Wellcome Australasia
53 Phillips Street
Concord
N.S.W. 2137
Australia

Miles Laboratories Aust. Ltd.
Wellington Road
Mulgrave
Victoria 3170
Australia

**Special Equipment Associated with Glomerular Culture**

Lab-Tek Culture Equipment
Miles Laboratories Inc.
P.O. Box 2000
Elkart, Ind. 46515

Falcon Flasks
Falcon Plastics
Los Angeles, Calif. 90061

Photo-Optical Data Analyser
L.W. International
Woodland Hills, Maine 04694

Cine-Microphotographic Equipment
Bolex
Sainte-Croix
Switzerland

Miles Laboratories Aust. Ltd.
Wellington Road
Mulgrave
Victoria 3170
Australia

**Optical Microscopes and Accessories**

Carl Zeiss Inc.
444 Fifth Avenue
New York, N.Y. 10018

E. Leitz Co.
468 Park Avenue South
New York, N.Y. 10016

Carl Zeiss
31 Foley Street
London W1P 8AP
England

E. Leitz Instruments Ltd.
30 Mortimer Street
London W1P 8AP
England

Olympus Optical Co. Ltd.
43-2, Hatagaya Zchome
Shibuya-Ku, Tokyo
Japan

C. Reichert Ltd.
Hernalser Hauptstrasse 219
A-1171
Wein
Austria

## Optical Microscopes and Accessories (continued)

Carl Zeiss Aust. Pty. Ltd.
396 Neerim Road
Carnegie
Victoria 3163
Australia

Olympus (Australian agents)
Anax Pty. Ltd.
147 Cardigan Street
Carlton
Victoria 3053
Australia

Reichert (Australian agents)
Selby Scientific Ltd.
352 Ferntree Gully Road
Notting Hill
Victoria 3168
Australia

Wild Leitz Aust. Pty. Ltd.
83 Palmerston Crescent
South Melbourne
Victoria 3205
Australia

## Electron Microscopes

AEI Scientific Apparatus Inc.
Kratos
4075 Ruffin Road
San Diego, Calif. 92123

Carl Zeiss Inc.
444 Fifth Avenue
New York, N.Y. 10018

Hitachi (U.S. agents)
Perkin Elmer Corporation
Instruments Division
Main Avenue
Norwalk, Conn. 06956

JEOL
477 Riverside Avenue
Bedford, Mass. 02155

Philips Electronics Instruments
750 South Fulton Avenue
Mount Vernon, N.Y. 10550

Siemens of America, Inc.
350 Fifth Avenue
New York, N.Y. 10001

AEI Scientific Apparatus Ltd.
Barton Dock Road
Urmston
Manchester M31 2LD
England

Carl Zeiss
31 Foley Street
London W1P 8AP
England

Hitachi (U.K. agents)
Perkin Elmer Ltd.
Post Office Lane
Beaconsfield
Buckinghamshire HP9 1QA
England

JEOL
Grove Park
Colindale
London N.W.9
England

Philips (U.K. agents)
Pye Unicam Ltd.
York Street
Cambridge CB1 2PX
England

Siemens U.K. Ltd.
Great West House
Great West Road
Brentford
Middlesex TW8 9DG
England

Carl Zeiss
7082 Oberkochen
West Germany

**Electron Microscopes (continued)**

Hitachi Ltd.
Naka Works
Katsuta, Ibaraki
Japan

JEOL
148 Nakagami Akishima
Tokyo 196
Japan

N. V. Philips
Gloeilampenfabrieken
Eindhoven
Netherlands

Siemens Aktiengesellschaft
Wernewerk fur Messtechnik
7500 Karlsruhe 21
Rheinbruchestrasse 50
West Germany

GEC Automation and Control (AEI)
660 Burwood Road
Hawthorn
Victoria 3122
Australia

Carl Zeiss Aust. Pty. Ltd.
396 Neerim Road
Carnegie
Victoria 3163
Australia

Hitachi (Australian agents)
N.I.C. Instrument Co.
Essendon Airport
North Essendon
Victoria 3041
Australia

Philips Scientific and Industrial
Equipment
153 Sturt Street
South Melbourne
Victoria 3205
Australia

JEOL
17 Villiers Place
Dee Why
N.S.W. 2099
Australia

Siemens Industries Ltd.
544 Church Street
Richmond
Victoria 3121
Australia

# INDEX

## F



## G

## O



## P



## R



## S

## T



## U



## V



## W